The Evaluation and Treatment of Eating Disorders

The Evaluation and Treatment of Eating Disorders

Diane Gibson, MS, OTR
Editor

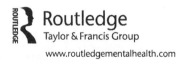

Routledge
Taylor & Francis Group

www.routledgementalhealth.com

The Evaluation and Treatment of Eating Disorders has also been published as *Occupational Therapy in Mental Health,* Volume 6, Number 1, Spring 1986.

The Haworth Press, Inc., 28 East 22 Street, New York, NY 10010-6194
EUROSPAN/Haworth, 3 Henrietta Street, London WC2E 8LU England

Library of Congress Cataloging in Publication Data

Main entry under title:

The Evaluation and treatment of eating disorders.

   Has also been published as: Occupational therapy in mental health,
v. 6, no. 1, spring 1986.
   Includes bibliographies.
   1. Appetite disorders—Addresses, essays, lectures. 2. Anorexia nervosa—Addresses, essays, lectures. 3. Occupational therapy—Addresses, essays, lectures. I. Gibson, Diane.
[DNLM: 1. Anorexia Nervosa—rehabilitation. 2. Appetite Disorders—rehabilitation.
3. Occupational Therapy. W1 OC601N v.6 no. 1/2/WM 175 E92]
RC552.A72E93   1986   616.85'2   85-24856
ISBN 0-86656-541-8

The Evaluation and Treatment of Eating Disorders

Occupational Therapy in Mental Health
Volume 6, Number 1

CONTENTS

When Doing Is Not Enough: The Relationship Between Activity and Effectiveness in Anorexia Nervosa   137

M. A. McColl, BSc, MHSc
J. Friedland, BA, MA, OT(C)
A. Kerr, BSc (OT)

Foreword

Eating disorders, including anorexia nervosa and bulimia, have become increasingly prevalent in hospitalized patient populations. However, few publications presently exist in occupational therapy literature. This issue addresses current interdisciplinary thinking regarding the theories, the evaluation, and the treatment of this pernicious syndrome.

Dr. David Waltos, in "Historical Perspectives and Diagnostic Considerations", describes the historical evolution of anorexia nervosa from the 1600's when it was noted as "a nervous atrophy caused by violent passions of the mind, intemperate drinking of spirituous liquors, and unwholesome air" to the 1980's when it has become recognized as a complex syndrome affecting psychological, physiological, and behavioral systems. Criteria for diagnosing anorexia nervosa are reviewed from the Diagnostic and Statistical Manual of Mental Disorders (DSM-III). Differential diagnosis is an important consideration in providing appropriate treatment, since other gastrointestinal, endocrine, and central nervous system diseases may mimic symptoms of anorexia nervosa.

In their article, "Behavioral Treatment of Eating Disorders", Kathleen and James McGee outline the history, theoretical assumptions, and prime methodologies of behavior therapy. After providing this conceptual background, they discuss etiology and treatment from a behavior modification frame of reference. Conditioned fear responses to various foods cause the anorexic patient to experience intense anxiety upon seeing or thinking about food. External reinforcers, such as family attention riveted on a starving young woman in conjunction with cultural emphasis on thinness, become powerful motives in stimulating and maintaining an emaciated state. Deprivation, contingency plans, informational feedback, and negative reinforcement are elements viewed as efficacious in treatment.

In an interesting discussion in "Treatment of the Hospitalized Eating Disordered Patient", of predispositional, precipitating, and perpetuating determinants, Dr. Roth, traces cultural, social, experiential, and somatic dimensions. The development of irrational self-beliefs in the premorbid anorexic patient allows her to set unrealistically high expectations at the same time she devalues her achievements and self-worth. Diet, exercise, and weight gain become measures of self-worth and are utilized to ward off panic about helplessness in an overcontrolling and overprotective family.

Milieu and treatment groups described by Dr. Roth are integrated into a multidisciplinary team effort. Supervision of eating, skill deficiencies, behavioral excesses, and cognitive functioning are primary foci in the highly structured treatment program.

Nancy Alexander, in her paper, "Characteristics and Treatment of Families with Anorectic Offspring", reviews material of family systems theorists noting their emphasis on the family's communication patterns, its leadership, and family roles and functions and beliefs of psychoanalytically oriented theorists who emphasize the personal qualities of family members and focus on the impact of parents on children in the family. This author provides insight into characteristics of families regularly producing anorexic offspring by charting three families' traits, communications, structure, and interpersonal transactions. She methodically compares and contrasts findings about these families against those identified by the theorists. Useful therapeutic interventions in the treatment of the family with anorectic children are discussed throughout the paper.

The articles written by occupational therapists are an excellent and significant beginning in the application of occupational therapy theory and practice to the treatment of eating disorders. Giles and Allen, in "Occupational Therapy in the Rehabilitation of the Patient with Anorexia Nervosa", review the prevailing theories of causation, then state that the occupational therapist's expertise in rehabilitation and analysis of functional abilities places him/her in an excellent position to assess and treat psychosocial dysfunction. Low self-esteem and a sense of powerlessness in the family underlie anorexic patients' needs to improve self-image and gain control in her environment. Therapeutic activities which help the anorexic patient to develop skill and pleasure in cooking, social activities, and leisure pursuits are fundamental. Expressive art therapy and movement therapy are also seen as significant in assisting the anorexic patient in identifying and in accepting her feelings. Cognitive behavior therapy is stressed, yet the approach is integrated with behavior therapy.

Roann Barris addresses the application of the model of human occupation to the treatment of eating disorders in her paper, "Occupational Dysfunction and Eating Disorders: Theory and Approach to Treatment.'' She reviews this relatively new occupational therapy theory, noting that eating disordered individuals demonstrate dysfunction in meaningful occupation as well as in weight control. Anorexic persons are characterized by struggling to attain personal control, an important component in personal causation which along with values and interests comprise the volition subsystem in the model. Values are determined by mass media and an overinvolved, protective family; and interests although initially broad based, frequently narrow to food preoccupation and a dearth of social and leisure activities.

In the habituation subsystem, the two components, habits and roles, are both pathologically affected. The anorexic girl tends to overly internalize the family role at the expense of other roles, such as worker or friend. Habits regarding food are ritualized and rigidly carried out. The performance subsystem encompasses perceptual-motor processes, interpersonal skills, and neurological or musculo-skeletal components, all of which may be present in the hospitalized anorexic patient.

Throughout this complex, yet clearly written article, the author compares and contrasts anorexia nervosa with bulimia. She identifies assessment scales and tests with which to evaluate components of the human occupation model as well as potential treatment activities.

Mary K. Bailey describes a comprehensive activity therapy program and a specialized eating disorders subprogram in her paper, ''Occupational Therapy for Patients with Eating Disorders''. Assessment procedures are oriented toward cognitive, motor, social, and self-concept areas as well as interdependent living skills, leisure skills, and work skills.

Bailey's assessments substantiate other reports in this issue, namely that anorexic patients demonstrate little awareness of their own values and leisure needs; they suffer from dramatically lowered self-esteem; their group interactional skills are uniformly diminished; and they are reluctant to involve themselves in tasks they cannot control.

Patients are scheduled in treatment groups on an individualized basis. Protocols of some groups are included in the article. Activities found to be beneficial include assertive communications, ceramics, leatherwork, weight training, dance therapy, art therapy, vocational counseling, and leisure community experiences. Excellent case histories which exemplify the symptomatology and treatment methodologies are presented.

A final paper entitled, "When Doing is not Enough: the Relationship Between Activity and Effectiveness" by McColl, Friedland, and Kerr identifies the core of anorexia nervosa as being a "pervasive sense of ineffectiveness" and a subsequent lack of personal identity. A specific hospital treatment regime is outlined in which privileges, such as unlimited activities, are contingent on weight gain. An occupational therapy assumption regarding positive correlation between successful completion of activities and a perceived sense of effectiveness is challenged. Anorexic patients do not feel pleasure and mastery from performing excellently. As in Barris' paper of human occupation, personal causation and ability to influence outcomes is an important experience in developing a healthy view of one's interactions with the environment, but unfortunately, not one available to the incipient anorexic individual. The subjective belief in one's competence is as significant as the objective capacity for success.

This paper also explores the history of activity analysis in occupational therapy, and its summary statement suggests that a less intuitive, more empirical conceptualization is needed before the meaning of activity can be understood and prescribed for specific patient groups, such as the eating disordered patient. Implications for treatment of the anorexic patient include allowing her to explore her environment and choose her own activity rather than prescribing it for her.

These articles represent an outstanding collection of interdisciplinary vantage points and overlapping theories as well as programmatic applications which should have immense value to the front-line clinician.

Diane Gibson, MS, OTR
Editor

The Evaluation and Treatment of Eating Disorders

Historical Perspectives
and Diagnostic Considerations

David L. Waltos, MD

ABSTRACT. From its first clear description in the late 17th century, the concept of anorexia nervosa has undergone numerous descriptive and ideologic changes, culminating in the present diagnostic classification which includes weight loss, disturbed body image, fear of obesity and refusal to maintain body weight in the absence of physical illness. Numerous associated clinical features are described, thereby aiding the assessment of the magnitude of the disorder and the development of an integrated treatment program. A differential diagnosis is presented.

INTRODUCTION

Although anorexia nervosa, as a separate disease entity, is approaching its 300th birthday, it remains an enigmatic and often times recalcitrant illness. Despite the many studies which have attempted to elucidate accurate descriptions, epidemiology, etiology and treatment protocols, it still remains one of the few psychiatric illnesses which can be unremitting until death. An historical overview demonstrates how present understanding is the culmination of an evolutionary process of additions and refinements, resulting in the criteria enumerated in the third edition of the *Diagnostic and Statistical Manual of Mental Disorders* (DSM III). A myriad of features, including psychological, behavioral and physiological concomitants further characterize the disorder, and although not necessary to make the diagnosis, have implications for better understanding the patient and planning an integrated treatment approach. Because of the complex multi-system effects of anorexia nervosa, its presentation can mimic many other illnesses. A comprehensive dif-

David L. Waltos is Admissions Officer at The Sheppard and Enoch Pratt Hospital, Towson, Maryland 21204.

1

ferential diagnosis must be reviewed to ensure that appropriate therapies are instituted.

HISTORY

The first detailed descriptions of anorexia nervosa were given by Sir Richard Morton (1689). He called it "a nervous atrophy", and clearly distinguished it from consumption, thereby recognizing the psychic influences which led to the act of self starvation:

> A nervous atrophy, or consumption, is a wasting of the body without any remarkable fever, cough or shortness of breath; but it is attended with a want of appetite, and a bad digestion upon which there follows a languishing weakness of nature, and a falling away of the flesh every day more and more . . . The causes which dispose the patient to this disease, I have for the most part observed to be violent passions of the mind, the intemperate drinking of spirituous liquors, and an unwholsom air, by which it is no wonder if the tone of the nerves and the temper of the spirits are destroyed.
>
> This distemper, as most other nervous diseases, is chronical, but very hard to be cured unless a physician be called at the beginning of it. At first it flatters and deceives the patient for which reason it happens for the most part that the physician is consulted too late. And at last it terminates in a hydropical and oedamatous swelling of the body, especially of the lower and depending parts, in which case there remain no hope of the patient's life, neither is there anything more to be done for his cure, than giving him some ease, whereby his miserable life may be lengthened for some days. (Morton, 1694)

His most famous case history follows:

> Mr. Duke's daughter in S. Mary Axe, in the year 1684 and the eighteenth year of her age, in the month of July fell into a total suppression of her monthly courses from a multitude of cares and passions of her mind but without any symptom of the green-sickness following upon it. From which time her appetite began to abate, and her digestion to be bad; her flesh also began to be flaccid and loose and her looks pale, with other symptoms usual in an universal consumption of the habit of the body . . .

I do not remember that I did ever in all my practice see one that was conversant with the living so much wasted with the greatest degree of consumption, (like a skeleton only clad with skin) yet there was no fever, but on the contrary, a coldness of the whole body; no cough, or difficulty with breathing, nor an appearance of any other distemper of the lungs, or of any other entrail; no looseness or any other sign of a colliquation, or pre-ternatural expence of the nutritious juices. Only her appetite was diminished, and her digestion uneasy, with fainting-fitts, which did frequently return upon her. (Morton, 1694)

It was not until 200 years later, when Sir William Gull (1868) in England and Dr. Charles Lasegue (1873) in France simultaneously, yet independently published their detailed medical reports, that interest was again rekindled in this enigmatic disease. Gull first mentioned it as a "hysteric apepsia" in an address at Oxford in 1868 but later coined the term "anorexia nervosa" (Gull, 1874). Lasegue named the illness "anorexie hysterique", a term still used in French-speaking countries. Interestingly, both are misnomers, as loss of appetite is not present until the later stages of the disorder, nor is it felt at present to be a hysterical condition. Nonetheless, the two authors provided excellent descriptions, recognized an emotional etiology, and described treatment not unlike our present regimens, including separation from family, rest, nourishment and supportive therapy. More importantly, Gull and Lasegue ushered in a century of descriptive and theoretical research which has further expanded our understanding of this complicated disorder. Numerous treatises appeared in England and France and finally in the United States where the American translation of Dejerine and Gauckler's *Psychoneurosis and Their Treatment by Psychotherapy* stated;

. . . every time that you find that the patient has gone upon a restricted diet, either voluntary or from some emotional cause and this has been followed by a loss of the psychic idea of appetite, you can safely assume the existence of mental anorexia. (Dejerine and Gauckler, 1913)

In 1914 Simmonds, a pathologist at the University of Hamburg, noted a necrotic pituitary in a woman who died of emaciation (Simmonds, 1914). This provided what appeared to be a ready explanation for many causes of extreme weight loss, and reports of "Simmonds' cachexia" flourished. Unfortunately it was used to label emaciation even in the absence of overt signs of pituitary failure, and it was not until later that Berkman (1930) and Venables (1930) separately "rediscovered" anorexia as a unique entity, noting not only that it was secondary to psychological disturbance, but also that many of the physiologic findings were reversible upon remission. Escamilla and Lisser (1942) reviewed the literature on Simmonds' disease, and found that only one sixth of cases were pathologically proven. What followed was an acceptance of anorexia nervosa and Simmonds' disease as separate entities, but only after many years of inappropriate diagnosis and treatment.

A trend toward diagnostic overgeneralization characterized the next twenty years, with numerous reports suggesting that the syndrome was nonspecific and broad. Bliss and Branch (1960) felt that a 25 pound weight loss, which could be attributed to a psychological cause, was the only necessary criterion to make the diagnosis! Hilda Bruch's contributions, starting in 1961, were a major factor in redirecting our thinking towards a more specific conceptualization (Bruch, 1962, 1965). She described a series of patients in which she found: 1) a disturbance in body image, 2) a failure to recognize nutritional needs, and 3) a pervasive sense of ineffectiveness. She also ushered in the concept of differential diagnosis, separating patients with true anorexia from those with similar manifestations secondary to other neurotic or schizophrenic disorders (Bruch, 1973). Selvini Palazzoli (1963, 1967) added still further clarifications along these lines, emphasizing the patient's attempts at gaining independence. At the same time a more behavioral framework was proposed by Crisp (1967) who believed that anorexia nervosa represented a weight phobia coupled with the fear of normal pubertal body development, while Russell (1969) believed the causation to be hypothalamic dysfunction, thereby disturbing the mechanisms regulating control of food intake. Extensive research has continued along all these lines, with over 100 new articles appearing each year.

DIAGNOSIS

Dependable diagnostic criteria are of paramount importance, not only for the purposes of conducting and evaluating the research noted above, but also for preventing the diagnosis from being made simply on the basis of exclusion of other "organic" causes. The first widely accepted inter-institutional criteria were published by Feighner et al. (1972), and are shown in Table 1. This standardization was a boon to diagnosis for both research and treatment purposes and prompted the American Psychiatric Association (1980) to

Table 1.

Feighner Criteria for Anorexia Nervosa

I.   Age at onset less than 25 years

II.   Accompanying weight loss of at least 25% of original body weight

III.   A distorted, implacable attitude toward eating, food, or weight that overrides hunger, admonitions, reassurance, and threats

    A.   Denial of illness, with a failure to recognize nutritional needs

    B.   Apparent enjoyment in losing weight, with overt manifestation that food refusal is a pleasurable indulgence

    C.   A desired body image of extreme thinness, with overt evidence that it is rewarding to the patient to achieve and maintain that state

    D.   Unusual hoarding or handling of food

IV.   No known medical illness that could account for the disorder and weight loss

V.   No other known psychiatric disorder, particulary primary affective disorders, schizophrenia, and obsessive-compulsive and phobic neuroses (the assumption is made than even though it may appear phobic or obsessional, food refusal alone is not sufficient to qualify for obsessive-compulsive or phobic disease)

IV.   Manifestation of at least two of:

    A.   Amenorrhea

    B.   Lanugo hair

    C.   Bradycardia (persistent resting pulse of 60 or less)

    D.   Periods of overactivity

    E.   Episodes of bulimia

    F.   Vomiting (may be self-induced)

Note.   From "Diagnostic Criteria for use in psychiatric research" by J.P. Feighner, E. Robins, S.B. Guze, R.A. Woodruff Jr., and G. Winokur, 1972, <u>Archives of General Psychiatry</u>, <u>26</u>, 57-63.

publish their now widely accepted scheme (Table 2). Although psychiatrists describe patients according to these criteria, they still clinically depend on Russell's triad of 1) self induced starvation, 2) morbid fear of fat and 3) an abnormality in hormonal functioning (amenorrhea in females; decreased sexual function in males) to guide them in their diagnostic interview (Russell, 1973; Anderson, 1985). The appropriate questions include: "Are you afraid that if you started eating normally, you would have no control over it, or wouldn't be able to stop?" or "Are you afraid of getting fat if you ate three meals per day?" Responses suggesting the fear of obesity in the presence of significant weight loss and amenorrhea (or decreased sexual interest in males) allows one to make the diagnosis with confidence. The numerous associated clinical features can be divided into three groups: behavioral, psychological and medical. They are not officially required to make the diagnosis, nor are some of them specific to anorexia nervosa, since they can be seen in normal individuals subject to food deprivation and are reversible upon weight gain. Their value lies in assisting the clinician in ruling out other illnesses (medical), understanding the patient more accurately (psychological), and devising an effective contingency-oriented treatment program (behavioral).

Table 2.

DSM III Criteria for Diagnosis of Anorexia Nervosa

A.   Intense fear of becoming obese, which does not diminish as weight loss progresses.

B.   Disturbance of body image, e.g. claiming to "feel fat" even when emaciated.

C.   Weight loss of at least 25% of original body weight or, if patient is under 18 years of age, weight loss from original body weight plus projected weight gain expected from growth charts may be combined to make the 25%.

D.   Refusal to maintain body weight over a minimal normal weight for age and height.

E.   No known physical illness that would account for the weight loss.

Note.   From Diagnostic & statistical manual of mental disorders, (3rd ed.) (p.69) by Psychiatric Association, 1980, Washington, D.C.: Author

I. Behavioral

Most commonly, one sees unusual behavior associated with food. These individuals often cook meals but refuse to eat them, or may in fact avoid eating in front of other people. Hoarding and concealing food, perhaps a result of the effects of starvation, are accompanied by secretive isolated meals, usually candy or foods high in carbohydrates. One may also see crumbling and/or throwing away of unconsumed foods. Excessive exercising, of ritual dimensions and inappropriate to the environment such as a very hot day, is invariably seen and includes bicycling, walking and push-ups. Intense mirror gazing and frequent weigh-ins reflect the patient's constant preoccupation with body size. Laxative and diuretic abuse is not infrequent, and compulsive stealing of candy or laxatives has also been observed. Socially, individuals regress to a more immature "prepubertal" pattern (Anderson, 1985). Dating ceases, as does contact with close friends. There is a markedly decreased interest in or abhorrence of sexual relations, and this is often accompanied by a heightened dependency on and compliance with parents, except over issues of food intake.

II. Psychological

Fears of fatness and weight gain pervade the anorectic patient's thinking. This may literally be their only experience, although some do feel pleasure and satisfaction as weight is lost. Denial of the illness is common and is accompanied by an over-estimation of the size of body parts. This perceptual distortion, which can be of delusional proportions, has been the subject of much discussion. Casper (1979) noted that it correlated directly with the severity of the illness, whereas others have been more specific, believing it to be related to the degree of vomiting (Button et al., 1977) or the degree of denial (Crisp and Kalucy, 1974). Unfortunately, normal age matched controls also overestimate; hence, its significance in anorexia is unclear. Symptoms directly attributable to starvation include intrusive thoughts and dreams about food and/or eating, as well as a generalized listless mental state (Anderson, 1985). Psychological testing often reveals these individuals to be of average intelligence, somewhat introverted, highly self-critical and prone to using an intellectual rather than a feeling perspective (Smart, et al., 1976). Their ability to tolerate emotions is characterized by restriction and over-control. The Rorschach Test reveals aggressively-colored answers especially of an oral character, such as engulfing figures (Theilgaard, 1965). The Thematic Apperception Test may show an infantile dependent attitude especially towards parents, or a mother fixation marked by ambivalence and/or guilt (Theilgaard, 1965).

Anxiety, depression and phobic or obsessional traits may be present. They are not specific to the illness, but if of sufficient magnitude may warrant additional diagnoses (Borderline Personality, Major Depression, etc.).

III. Medical

Starvation brings with it a multitude of manifestations. There is a marked loss of fat and muscle tissue giving the patient the appearance of a concentration camp victim. Urination may increase, heart rate and respirations are slowed, and blood pressure drops. With severe weight loss, body temperature may go as low as 35 °C, and dependent edema and lanugo (neonatal-like hair) appear.

Many hormonal changes take place, and in many female patients the resulting amenorrhea actually precedes weight loss. Studies of luteinizing hormone (LH) secretion reveal that it is similar to that in prepubertal females, and that levels of both LH and estrogen are markedly diminished in emaciation (Halmi, 1978). Although this normalizes with weight gain, it does not guarantee the return of menses, thus implying that other factors may play a role in the prolonged amenorrhea seen in some women. Other hormonal changes include low amounts of thyroid hormones (Alexander, et al., 1964; Chopra and Smith, 1975), normal or elevated growth hormone levels (Frankel and Jenkins, 1975), decreased testosterone in males (Boyar and Bradlow, 1977), and incomplete suppression of ACTH and cortisol by dexamethasone (Halmi, 1975). The dexamethasone suppression test cannot be used to support the diagnosis, as positive test results are seen in many other illnesses. Routine laboratory tests often reveal the presence of anemia, low numbers of white cells with a preponderance of lymphocytes and decreased levels of fibrinogen (used for blood clotting), all of which normalize with weight gain. Liver function tests, the electrocardiogram and the electroencephalogram can all be abnormal. Hypercarotenemia, which gives the skin an orange tinge, is reversible with weight gain (Dally, 1959).

In addition to the effects of starvation, methods used to induce weight loss lead to complications. vomiting and purging cause potassium levels to drop and can lead not only to cardiac arrhythmias, but also to death secondary to cardiac arrest. Seizures and tetany can result from the metabolic imbalance caused by low potassium levels, but overt peripheral neuropathies are rare (Anderson, 1985). Acid content of the vomitus erodes tooth enamel, thus causing decay and other dental complications. Laxative abuse can lead to chronic constipation and episodic diarrhea. Epigastric and/or abdominal discomfort is common, and gastric dilatation can be a rare complication (Halmi, 1975).

EPIDEMIOLOGY

The age of onset is typically described as being from late adolescence to the early thirties, with the ages of 12 to 18 being considered high risk (American Psychiatric Association, 1980). This disorder occurs predominantly in females (95%) (American Psychiatric Association, 1980, Halmi, 1974) and appears to be more common in middle and upper classes as well as in professions that demand the maintenance of low weight such as models, actresses, ballet dancers, flight attendants and jockeys (Anderson, 1985). Precipitating factors are very difficult to identify, although events such as normal dieting or comments about the person's increasing weight have been implicated. The incidence (number of new cases per year) had been estimated at .37 per 100,000 (Kendall et al., 1973), and may be on the increase (Theander, 1970). Many centers report treating larger numbers of these patients, although this may be secondary to earlier or better recognition rather than an increase in the numbers per se. The prevalence (or number of cases at any given time) is estimated at 1% of middle class adolescent girls (Andersen, 1985). Possible hereditary transmission of this disorder has been raised by the occurrence of this illness in twins, siblings and mother child pairs (Lucas, 1981). Kalucy et al. (1977) showed 16% of mothers and 23% of fathers of anorectic patients had a history in adolescence of low weight or weight phobia. However the frequency of these associations is extremely low and has not been studied systematically. Family characteristics—enmeshment, rigidity, overprotectiveness and poor conflict resolution—have been implicated in the genesis of this disorder (Rosman et al., 1977). However, many seemingly normal families also contain anorectic individuals, so the significance of these findings remain unproven.

The course runs the gamut from spontaneous recovery without treatment, episodes of weight gain followed by relapses, to death despite treatment from the complications of starvation. Most commonly, a single episode is followed by full recovery (American Psychiatric Association, 1980). A good prognostic indicator is early age of onset, whereas poor prognostic indicators are later age of onset and a high number of prior hospitalizations (Halmi, 1975). Short term response to hospital-based treatment programs is good (Halmi, 1975) but relapses or a transition to bulimia may occur (Andersen, 1985). The mortality rate had been between 15 and 21% (American Psychiatric Association, 1980), but many series now report rates of 0-2% (Andersen, 1985), most likely because of earlier identification and referral to experienced treatment teams.

DIFFERENTIAL DIAGNOSIS

The differential diagnosis encompasses both psychiatric and medical disorders. Most other illnesses can be ruled out by taking an adequate history and mental status examination, inquiring not only about the features of anorexia nervosa, but also about the associated concomitants of other disorders under consideration. Laboratory evaluations should be specific and only used to further refine complex diagnostic dilemmas.

Medical illnesses include gastrointestinal (malabsorption, ulcers, irritable bowel syndromes), endocrine (Addison's Disease, hyperthyroidism, hypopituitarism, diabetes), and central nervous system (hypothalamic tumor) pathology. Panhypopituitarism (Simmonds' Disease) had obviously been confused with anorexia nervosa. However, it usually occurs in middle age and is precipitated by physical illness. The lassitude and weakness seen in this disease (as well as Addison's disease and diabetes) is quite uncommon in anorexia. Carcinoma, especially gastrointestinal, can mimic many symptoms of this disorder, as can tuberculosis and regional enteritis. However, these patients lack confirmation by DSM III criteria, although judicious use of laboratory tests and radiography may be necessary to establish a definitive diagnosis.

Of the psychiatric illnesses, depression with weight loss may be confused with anorexia nervosa. However, in pure depression, fear of obesity is absent, appetite is decreased and the agitation is not the planned ritualistic activity seen in anorexia. The two syndromes can co-exist, in which case both diagnoses should be made. Somatization disorders must also be considered, although fear of obesity is absent, the weight loss is less severe, and amenorrhea rarely lasts longer than three months. Schizophrenia with delusions about food is relatively easy to discern because of impaired reality testing in other spheres, and the delusions are seldom concerned with the food's caloric content.

Bulimia, as defined by binges followed by depression, self deprecating thoughts and vomiting, is recognized as a separate syndrome, although it can co-exist with anorexia nervosa. Weight is usually maintained in bulimia, or if it is lost, it is never as great as 25% of the body weight. Nonetheless, the associated features of these two disorders are so similar that one should not be considered without the other. Lastly, psychogenic dysphasia, globus hystericus ("lump in the throat") and drug use, including amphetamines, cocaine and diet pills, should be considered. The importance of careful history taking cannot be overestimated.

SUMMARY

Although anorexia nervosa is a relatively rare disease and has not been readily accessible for study, much has been learned about the clinical symptomatology. At no time in its 300 year history has diagnostic acumen been as refined as it is today, yet there are still large gaps in our available knowledge. There are no definitive genetic data, nor are causative factors clear. An integration of psychodynamic, physiologic, behavioral and family-oriented paradigms may lead to the best model for assessment and treatment (Lucas, 1981), but more research is necessary. Only through better long term follow-up studies can we gain a more thorough understanding of this illness, with the eventual goal of early identification and prevention of a serious disease of the times.

REFERENCES

Alexander, W. D., Harrison, M. T., Harden, R. McC., & Koutras, D. A. (1964). The effects of total fasting on thyroid function in man. *Metabolism, 19*, 587-590.

American Psychiatric Association. (1980). *Diagnostic and statistical manual of mental disorders* (3rd ed.). Washington, DC: Author.

Andersen, A. E. (1985). *Practical comprehensive treatment of anorexia nervosa and bulimia*. Baltimore: Johns Hopkins University Press.

Berkman, J. M. (1930). Anorexia nervosa, anorexia, inanition, and low based metabolic rate. *American Journal of Medical Science, 180*, 411-424.

Bliss, E. L., & Branch, C. H. H. (1960). *Anorexia nervosa: its history, psychology and biology*. New York: Paul B. Hoeber.

Boyar, R. M., & Bradlow, H. L. (1977). Studies of testosterone metabolism in anorexia nervosa. In R. A. Vigersky (Ed.), *Anorexia Nervosa* (pp. 271-275). New York: Raven Press.

Bruch, H. (1962). Perceptual and conceptual disturbances in anorexia nervosa. *Psychosomatic Medicine, 24,* 187-194.

Bruch, H. (1965). Anorexia nervosa and its differential diagnosis. *Journal of Nervous and Mental Diseases, 141,* 555-566.

Bruch, H. (1973). *Obesity and anorexia nervosa.* New York: Basic Books.

Button, E. J., Fransella, F., & Slade, P. D. (1977). A reappraisal of body perception disturbance in anorexia nervosa. *Psychological Medicine, 7*(2), 235-243.

Cooper, R. C., Halmi, K. A., Goldberg, S. C., Eckert, E. D., & Davis, J. M. (1979). Disturbance in body image estimation as related to other characteristics and outcome in anorexia nervosa. *British Journal of Psychiatry, 134,* 60-66.

Chopra, I. J., & Smith, S. R. (1975). Circulating thyroid hormones and thyrotropin in adult patients with protein-calorie malnutrition. *Journal of Clinical Endocrinology and Metabolism, 40,* 221-227.

Crisp, A. H. (1967). The possible significance of some behavioral correlates of weight and carbohydrate intake. *Journal of Psychosomatic Research, 11,* 117-131.

Crisp, A. H., & Kalucy, R. S. (1974). Aspects of the perceptual disorder in anorexia nervosa. *British Journal of Medical Psychology, 47*(4), 349-361.

Dally, P. (1959). Carotenaemia occurring in a case of anorexia nervosa. *British Medical Journal, 5133,* 1333.

Dejerine, T., & Gauckler, E. (1913). *The psychoneuroses and their treatment by psychotherapy.* Philadelphia: J. B. Lippincott Co.

Escamilla, R. F., & Lisser, H. (1942). Simmonds' disease: a clinical study with review of the literature: differentiation from anorexia nervosa by statistical analysis of 595 cases, 101 of which were proven pathologically. *Journal of Clinical Endocrinology, 2,* 65-96.

Feighner, J. P., Robins, E., Guze, S. B., Woodruff, R. A., Jr., Winokur, G., & Munoz, R. (1972). Diagnostic criteria for use in psychiatric research. *Archives of Genreal Psychiatry, 26,* 57-63.

Frankel, R. J., & Jenkins, J. S. (1975). Hypothalamic pituitary function in anorexia nervosa. *Acta Endocrinologica, 78,* 209-221.

Gull, W. W. (1868). Address in medicine. *Lancet, 2,* 171-176.

Gull, W. W. (1874). Anorexia nervosa (apepsia hysterica, anorexia hysterica). *Transcripts of the Clinical Society of London, 7,* 22-28.

Halmi, K. A. (1974). Anorexia nervosa: demographic and clinical features in 94 cases. *Psychosomatic Medicine, 36,* 18-26.

Halmi, K. A. (1975). Anorexia nervosa. In H. I. Kaplan, A. M. Freedman, & B. J. Sadock (Eds.), *Comprehensive textbook of psychiatry/III: Vol. 2* (pp. 1882-1891). Baltimore: Williams and Wilkins.

Halmi, K. A. (1978). Anorexia nervosa: recent investigations. *Annual Review of Medicine, 29,* 137-148.

Kalucy, R. S., Crisp, A. H., & Harding, B. (1977). A study of 56 families with anorexia nervosa. *British Journal of Medical Psychology, 50*(4), 381-395.

Kendell, R. E., Hall, D. J., Harley, A., & Babigian, H. M. (1973). The epidemiology of anorexia nervosa. *Psychological Medicine, 3,* 200-203.

Lasegue, Charles (1873). On hysterical anorexia. *Medical Times Gazette, 2,* 265-266; 367-369.

Lucas, A. R. (1981). Toward an understanding of anorexia nervosa as a disease entity. *Mayo Clinic Proceedings, 56,* 254-264.

Morton, R. (1689). *Phthisiologica, seu exercitationes de phthisi tribus libris comprehensae: totumque opus variis historiis illustratum.* London: Samuel Smith.

Morton, R. (1694). *Phthisiologica: or, a treatise of consumptions.* London: Smith and Walford.

Rosman, B. L., Minuchin, S., Baker, L. & Leibman, R. (1977). A family approach to anorexia nervosa: study, treatment, and outcome. In R. A. Vigersky (Ed.), *Anorexia nervosa* (pp. 341-348). New York: Raven Press.

Russell, G. F. M. (1969). Metabolic, endocrine and psychiatric aspects of anorexia nervosa. *Scientific Basis of Medicine, Ann. Rev.*, 236-255.

Russell, G. F. M. (1973). The management of anorexia nervosa. In Royal College of Physicians of Edinburgh, *Symposium—anorexia nervosa and obesity* (Publication No. 42). Edinburgh: T. and A. Constable Ltd.

Selvini Palazzoli, M. (1963). *L'anoressia mentale*. Milano: Feltrinelli.

Selvini Palazzoli, M. (1967). La strutturazione della coscineze corporea, *Infanzia Anormale*, 73, 9-30.

Simmonds, M. (1914). Ueber hypophysisschwund mit tödlichem ausgang. *Deutsche Medizinische Wochenschrift, 40*, 322-323.

Smart, D., Beaumont, P., & George, G. (1976). Some personality characteristics of patients with anorexia nervosa. *British Journal of Psychiatry, 128*, 57-60.

Theander, S. (1970). Anorexia nervosa—a psychiatric investigation of 94 female patients. *Acta Psychiatrica Scananairca*, 214, (Suppl. 214).

Theilgaard, A. (1965). Psychological testing of patients with anorexia nervosa. In J. E. Meyer & H. Feldman (Eds.), *Gottingen* (p. 122). Stuttgart: Thieme.

Venables, J. F. (1930). Anorexia nervosa: a study of the pathogenesis and treatment of nine cases. *Guy Hospital Reports, 80*, 213-226.

Behavioral Treatment
of Eating Disorders

Kathleen T. McGee, BA
James P. McGee, PhD

ABSTRACT. Behavioral conceptualizations of anorexia nervosa and bulimia emphasize the notion that the symptoms of these disorders are acquired through processes of conditioning or learning. Behavioral therapy interventions have largely focused on reduction of the phobic-like anxiety associated with eating and weight gain, along with "reinforcement" of behaviors incompatible with pathological dieting. The results of follow-up research on the behavioral treatment of eating disorders are inconclusive; yet, most contemporary treatment "programs" for anorexia and bulimia involve at least limited use of behavior therapy principles.

DEFINITION OF BEHAVIOR THERAPY

Behavior therapy has been defined as "treatment deducible from the socio-psychological model that aims to alter a person's behavior directly through application of general psychological principles" (Ullmann and Krasner, 1966). Joseph Wolpe (1969), a pioneer in the development of behavior therapy, describes it as "the use of experimentally established principles of learning for the purpose of changing unadaptive habits." The earliest reference to behavior therapy in the professional literature appeared in 1953 in a monograph written by Lindsley, Skinner and Solomon which described the use of operant conditioning principles to alter behavior in regressed adult psychotics. There are presently at least a dozen or more definitions of behavior therapy, all of which share the following common features:

1. A focus on observable and directly measurable target behaviors;

Dr. McGee is Director of Psychology at The Sheppard and Enoch Pratt Hospital in Towson, Maryland 21204.

15

2. An effort to establish causal relationships between antecedents, behavior and consequences, particularly through the use of a "Skinnerian" experimental analysis of behavior; and
3. An emphasis on operational definition of concepts so that they can be replicated experimentally.

HISTORY

Shortly after the turn of the century, the Behavioral School of Psychology was established in the United States by John B. Watson, who many regard as the "Father of Modern Behaviorism." Watson's work, which was greatly influenced by the research of Pavlov on the conditioned reflex, involved the application of learning principles to alter behavior patterns in both animals and human subjects. In addition to Pavlov, Watson also fell under the influence of American psychologist E. L. Thorndike. Thorndike's "law of effect" which, in its simplest form, states that behavior is influenced by its consequences, provided the foundation for the behavioral psychology of operant conditioning which was developed by B. F. Skinner of Harvard University. Skinner's research on the systematic use of reward and punishment to influence behavior is generally regarded to be one of the major cornerstones of modern behavior therapy. Perhaps the two other most significant trends affecting the development of the field of behavior therapy were: the development of a learning theory model of psychopathology as a competing alternative to the disease or medical model; and a growing dissatisfaction, both among the lay public and the mental health professions, with the various psychodynamically-based psychotherapies because of their alleged inefficacy (Eysenck, 1952).

THEORETICAL ASSUMPTIONS OF BEHAVIOR THERAPY

The first and clearly most fundamental theoretical assumption upon which behavior therapy technologies are based is that human behavior is acquired through various processes of learning or conditioning. Behavior therapists make no distinction between the mechanisms by which adaptive or prosocial forms of behavior and maladaptive or deviant behaviors are learned. According to behavior therapists, just as one can learn how to play the piano or speak a particular language, so also can a person learn how to be pathologically aggressive, or in the case of anorexic patients, morbidly fearful of the prospect of gaining weight. Following from the pivotal assumption that all behavior, including behavior designated as pathological, is acquired through learning, it follows that in order to alter behavior, learning principles must be applied. There are essentially three processes of learning or behavioral acquisition that behavior therapists regard to be highly important. These are: classical or Pavlovian conditioning, operant or Skinnerian conditioning, and modeling or imitation learning.

Pavlovian conditioning, also known as classical or reflexive conditioning, is primarily related to the establishment of reflexive responses which are regulated by subcortical sections of the autonomic nervous system. In a typical early experiment, Pavlov would present a laboratory animal with some neutral stimulus, such as a tone, along with a stimulus such as food, which automatically elicited a salivatory response. Through repeated pairings of these two stimuli, Pavlov demonstrated that eventually the previously neutral stimulus, the tone, would ultimately elicit a salivatory response. Pavlov and other investigators went on to demonstrate that a broad array of responses, such as sweating, heart rate, gastrointestinal secretions, nausea, vomiting, tendon jerks, and limb withdrawal, could be conditioned to respond to stimuli which under normal circumstances would not produce such a response. Pavlov's research was conducted almost exclusively on animal subjects. However, in the early 1920's in this country, John Watson demonstrated that Pavlovian conditioning principles could also be applied to human subjects. Specifically, he was able to show that anxiety and phobic-like responses could be induced in human subjects by pairing neutral stimuli with aversive stimulation, such as a loud noise, which would cause a startle response. Although Watson's original experiments demonstrated the acquisition of anxiety responses under conditions of single exposure to intense aversive stimulation, other investigators have provided experimental evidence that phobic responses can also be developed after repeated exposure to mild levels of aversive stimulation. Joseph Wolpe, who stands out as a pioneer in the behavioral treatment of anxiety disorders, relies heavily on a Pavlovian model to both explain the acquisition of anxiety disorders and construct treatment interventions for their remediation.

The second major form of conditioning or learning felt to be important by behavior therapists is operant conditioning. Most of the early research on operant conditioning was also done with animals. In the typical experiment on this form of learning, an animal was confined in a small enclosure where his behavior could be directly altered by the systematic application of rewards and punishments. The famous "Skinner" box is one such version of this experimental apparatus. In one end of the Skinner box, there is a small lever which, when pressed by the animal, releases a food pellet reward accessible to the animal. An animal placed in such an apparatus can be quickly taught to perform complicated series of behaviors through the simple use of various types of reinforcement.

There are essentially four different types or categories of reinforcement that may follow a particular behavior. They are positive reinforcement, negative reinforcement, punishment, and the absence of reinforcement or extinction. Positive reinforcement involves the delivery of some type of reward or pleasurable stimulus contingent on the performance of a specific behavior. Positive reinforcement has the effect of increasing the probability of the recurrence of the behavior which preceded it. Negative reinforcement on the other hand involves the elimination of aversive stimulation contingent on the display of behavior. Both positive and negative reinforcement have the same effect, namely, increasing the recurrence of behavior in the future. Unlike negative reinforcement, punishment involves the direct application of aversive stimulation contingent on behavior so as to produce a termination or reduction in the targeted behavior. The consequences of no reinforcement or an extinction schedule are similar to those of punishment, namely, the suppression of behavior. Efforts to explain psychological deviancy in terms of operant conditioning have for the most part emphasized the notion that maladaptivity arises from a maladaptive reinforcement history. Seen this way, deviance is largely a form of social behavior composed of maladaptive operant responses. Furthermore, it is felt that well established deviant responses preclude the acquisition of more prosocial behavior.

At this point in time, practically all forms of social deviance and psychopathology have been treated through the use of operant conditioning principles. For example, the "token economy" has become a mainstay in the treatment armamentarium of mental health professionals involved in the rehabilitation of hospitalized schizophrenic patients.

Up until the mid-1960's, the literature on behavior therapy was dominated by descriptions of theoretical conceptualizations and behavioral procedures based almost exclusively on operant and classical conditioning. More recently, however, behaviorists have become interested in a third form of learning, namely, observational or imitation learning. Imitation learning quite simply refers to the fact that a wide array of human behaviors, both adaptive and maladaptive, have been acquired through a process of imitation. Here the "observer" watches a "model" perform some particular type of behavior and through the process of observation acquires the behavior himself. Most of the early research on observational learning was conducted by Albert Bandura and his associates (Bandura, Ross and Ross, 1963). In his studies on the acquisition of aggressive behavior in children, he demonstrated rather convincingly that aggressive behavior could quickly be acquired by children via the model-observer paradigm. As is the case with other forms of learning, the research on imitation indicates that misbehavior can be acquired through imitation just as readily as adaptive behavior can.

BEHAVIORAL CONCEPTUALIZATIONS OF EATING DISORDERS

Behavioral theories of the etiology of eating disorders typically involve an emphasis on all three forms of conditioning or learning. Anorexic and bulimic patients, for example, are thought to have a wide range of conditioned fear responses to various food, eating and weight gain stimuli that under normal conditions are affectively neutral. So, for example, when the anorexic patient sees food, thinks about food, or even prepares to enter the dining room, they experience intense, anxious arousal. The behavior therapist would argue that these anxiety responses are reflexive in nature and result from prior conditioning experiences. The avoidance and withdrawal behavior so characteristic of anorexic patients when they are exposed to food or an eating situation would be seen as operant behavior. The reinforcement for this operant withdrawal is a reduction in the anxiety feelings that occur when the anorexic is confronted with food or other eating stimuli. In addition, it is also posited that the starvation behavior of the anorexic receives powerful social reinforcement to the extent that the anorexic's behavior serves as an effective form of influence over other members of her social environment, particularly her parents. The emaciated appearance of a starving anorexic does, of course, normally elicit high levels of caring attention. This attention which is received contingent on the maladaptive behavior of self-imposed starvation is seen by behavior therapists as being a powerful motive for the maintenance of the behavior. Recently, the societal and cultural emphasis on slimness has been seen as a factor contributing to the current epidemic of eating disorders in this country. This cultural influence is most readily explained by behavior therapists through principles of imitation learning. Mainly, the anorexic patient is viewed as falling under the influence of socially sanctioned "models" of extreme thinness in the media and through advertising. Indeed, it is a rather common clinical occurrence to have anorexic patients report that television commercials and magazine ads promoting the cosmetic merits of slimness have had a powerful influence on their choice to engage in self-imposed starvation.

TREATMENT AND OUTCOME

As a treatment modality for anorexia nervosa, bulimia, and other eating disorders, behavior therapy is a relative newcomer. Prior to 1959, treatment for anorexia followed the traditional medical model, i.e., hospitalization, confinement to bed, supervised or forced feeding, traditional psychotherapy and/or family therapy (Agras and Kraemer, 1983).

However, in recent years, behavior therapy techniques have become almost a standard element in the treatment programs of hospitalized anorexic patients.

Behaviorally-oriented in-patient treatment programs typically include some or all of these elements:

1. Deprivation: Patients are given restricted access to such amenities as social contact, television, visits from friends and family, day-room privileges, telephone calls, exercise, etc.
2. Contingency plans: Access to the above-mentioned activities are linked to compliance with various aspects of the treatment plan (Halmi, Powers and Cunningham, 1975). For example, the patient may watch television when she has eaten so many meals or gained a predetermined amount of weight, etc. Halmi (1982) reports that the most effective behavioral programs are those that are individualized. Therapists may negotiate a treat-

ment contract with the patient which spells out the specific
system of reinforcements and reinforcement schedule. The patient herself may participate in the plan in that some studies
have enlisted the patient's input as to desirable reinforcers,
i.e., what would be most likely to motivate the patient to comply (Bhanji and Thompson, 1974, cited in Bemis, 1978).

3. Informational feedback: The patient is given precise and frequent informational feedback regarding the number of calories
   consumed and/or the amount of weight gained or lost.
   Sometimes the feedback is monitored by the patient herself,
   under supervision of the therapist, having the patient keep the
   charts and records of her own progress. Agras, Barlow,
   Chapin, Abel and Leitenberg (1974) report that feedback may
   be the most important variable in a behavioral treatment program in that it sets the occasion for reinforcement by inducing
   increased eating. In their series of single-case experiments
   designed to clarify the effectiveness of separate therapeutic
   variables, feedback and reinforcement seemed to be linked,
   and in the absence of feedback, positive reinforcement appeared to be relatively ineffective. The best results were obtained by a combination of feedback, reinforcement, and large
   meals.

4. Negative reinforcement: Most behavioral treatment programs
   involve an initial hospitalization. Agras, Barlow, Chapin, Abel
   and Leitenberg (1974) felt that negative reinforcement could
   play a part in weight gain, when discharge from the hospital
   was contingent upon weight gain. In one portion of their study,
   patients expressed a strong desire to get out of the hospital.
   Their cooperation with the program could have been an effort
   to avoid the unpleasant conditions of their hospital stay.

Most behavioral therapy programs seem strongly geared toward
the objective of weight gain, at least initially. And behavior therapy
seems to be most effective in the medical management and nutritional rehabilitation of the patient (Halmi, 1982). It has also been
reported to achieve a weight gain significantly faster than either
medical or drug therapy (Agras and Kraemer, 1983). Given that
long-term recovery will be discussed later, and can almost be
regarded as a separate issue (Argas, Stunkard and Blinder, 1974,
cited in Bemis, 1978), operant techniques have demonstrated a
remarkable facility in achieving the first critical step in treatment,

that of restoring weight (Bemis, 1978, Cinciripini, Kornblith, Turner, and Hersen, 1983).

An additional useful effect of behavioral treatment in a hospital setting was reported by Rosman, Bernice, Minuchin, et al., (in Vigersky, 1977). In this study, behavioral treatment was judged to be as useful in reducing confrontations as it was in reversing eating behavior.

Discussion of the long-term efficacy of behavior therapy in the treatment of anorexia nervosa necessitates the caveat that there have been very few controlled treatment studies and few, if any, of the follow-up studies that have been conducted have met ideal criteria (Halmi, 1983). There are several factors which may prejudice follow-up studies of cases where behavior therapy has been the initial method or the primary element of initial treatment of anorexics:

1. Whether or not behavior therapy was utilized as the post-discharge method of treatment.
2. What the age of onset and pre-treatment weights of the patients were. Since later age of onset, lower weight upon commencement of treatment, and longer duration of illness seem to be predictors of poor outcome (Halmi, 1982, Agras and Kraemer, 1983), these factors must be taken into account when judging the conclusions of follow-up research.
3. Size of patient sample: There are few studies which have included large numbers of patients and many which have included very few patients.
4. Length of follow-up: Some studies have reached conclusions after a relatively short follow-up time.
5. What criteria are used to determine outcome, i.e., does "cure" or "normal" include one, some, or all of the following considerations—weight gain, normalization of eating patterns, maintenance of normal weight, and psychosocial adjustment (Bemis, 1978, Pertschuk, cited in Vigersky, 1977).

Results of follow-up studies on the use of behavior therapy in the treatment of anorexia nervosa may be summarized under the following headings:

1. Studies which have found no difference in outcome between the use of behavior therapy and other therapies, or no therapy at all. A follow-up study reported by Bhanji and Thompson (Bemis, 1978), reporting on a relatively long follow-up period (32 months), con-

cludes that: "Operant conditioning techniques are often inadequate for long-term maintenance of normal eating habits and weight and are best used as a means of rapid weight restoration at times of nutritional crisis." A number of researchers conclude that long-term outcome depends more on factors relating to the severity of the illness rather than the method of treatment (Halmi, 1983). In a study reviewing treatments for anorexia over the last 50 years, Agras and Kraemer (1983) conclude that there is no difference between the effectiveness of behavior therapy, medical therapy, and drug therapy. This conclusion is tempered by the fact that, when medical therapy was exclusively used for treatment of anorexia, i.e., from 1930 till 1970, entry weights of patients were significantly higher than they have been during the last 20 years, when behavior and drug therapy began to be utilized. In a follow-up study of 27 cases, Pertschuk (cited in Vigersky, 1977) reported that, while a behaviorally-oriented hospital treatment was generally effective in helping patients gain weight, only two out of 25 patients could be said to be completely recovered upon follow-up and that improvement in the hospital was not predictive of long-term recovery. It must be noted that this study also included family, group, occupational, and recreation therapy while in hospital, and behavior therapy was *not* continued for the patients as a rule after discharge. Garfinkel (cited in Vigersky, 1977), upon review of 42 patients with a minimum follow-up period of one year, concluded that most patients improved regardless of the treatment method, and some patients fared poorly despite a variety of treatments.

2. Studies which support the continued use of behavior therapy after discharge from hospital: Agras and Kraemer (1983) report that, although the length of their follow-up was quite short, the superior efficacy of behavior therapy was sustained over time. Halmi, Powers and Cunningham (1975) have suggested that the effectiveness of behavior therapy for anorexia in hospital is maximized when it is continued after discharge.

3. Studies which recommend a combination of therapies as postdischarge treatment: Several researchers have concluded that a combination of treatment methods is the best course to follow in the treatment of anorexia. Halmi (1982) suggests that treatment must be multifaceted and should include medical management, personal, behavioral, and family therapies. In a study of 53 cases, with a median one-year follow-up, Rosman, Minuchin, Baker and Liebman (cited in Vigersky, 1977) report on a group of patients whose

hospital treatment used a behavioral paradigm, but the main emphasis both in and post-hospital was on a family approach. They report a success rate of 88%, in which symptoms disappeared two to eight weeks after treatment began. In a study on bulimia, Lacey (1982 cited in Johnson, Lewis and Hagman, 1984) reported on the use of a treatment method utilizing group therapy which moved gradually from behavioral strategies to insight-oriented treatment. In this controlled study, the control group showed no effect of treatment upon two-year follow-up, while the experimental group showed a 93% rate of remission.

4. Studies which suggest that weight gain upon follow-up may not mean a resolution of the eating disorder or a normal psychosocial adjustment of anorexic patients: Bemis (1978) states that the level of social and emotional adjustment achieved by the treated patient is frequently omitted from the limited follow-up information published, and when it is included, the apparent success rate may drop precipitously. In his follow-up study, Pertschuk (cited in Vigersky, 1977), concluded that a "good" adjustment did not necessarily imply resolution of the eating disorder. He reported that in his sample of patients, although weight may have increased, so did other eating abnormalities, e.g., bulimia developed in 10 of his 27 patients (none of the patients had bulimia on admisssion to the treatment program). He concluded that normalization of eating patterns did not parallel normalization of weight. Most of his patients at follow-up expressed an inordinate concern with food. However, he states that the in-hospital treatment program concentrated on weight gain and patients received little attention to eating patterns, nutrition, etc. Bemis (1978) suggests that the treatment techniques used thus far have not dealt with the conditions that maintain anorexic behavior in some individuals. She feels that researchers must deal with all the emotional and behavioral problems associated with anorexia nervosa.

A final issue which must be addressed is the contention of several therapists that behavioral treatment of anorexia nervosa can cause serious psychological damage to the patient. Bruch (1974) claims that the very efficiency of behavior modification increases the inner turmoil of patients and cited nine patients in whom she felt behavior therapy had undermined the patient's self-esteem and led to more serious psychological and eating problems. In contrast, while not claiming that behavior therapy is necessarily superior to other forms of treatment, several researchers have found that there is no evidence that behavior therapy is damaging to the anorectic patient

(Pertschuk, in Vigersky, 1977, Garfinkel, in Vigersky, 1977). Some behavioral therapists have responded to the criticisms by maintaining that, while weight loss is only one of the problems involved in anorexia, it is clearly the most critical (Agras, Stunkard and Blinder, 1974, cited in Bemis, 1978).

REFERENCES

Agras, W., Barlow, D., Chapin, H., Abel, G., Leitenberg, H. (1974). Behavior modification of anorexia nervosa. *Archives of General Psychiatry, 30,* 279-286.

Agras, W. S., & Kraemer, H. C. (1983). The treatment of anorexia nervosa: Do different treatments have different outcomes? *Psychiatric Annals, 13,* 928-935.

Bandura, A., Ross, D. & Ross, S. A. (1963). Imitation of Film Mediated Aggressive Models. *Journal of Abnormal and Social Psychology, 66,* 3-11.

Bemis, K. (1978). Current approaches to the etiology and treatment of anorexia nervosa. *Psychological Bulletin, 85,* 593-617.

Bruch, H. (1974). Perils of behavior modification in the treatment of anorexia nervosa. *Journal of the American Medical Association, 230,* 1419-1422.

Cinciripini, P., Kornblith, S., Turner, S., & Hersen, M. (1983). A behavioral program for the management of anorexia and bulimia. *Journal of Nervous and Mental Disease, 171,* 186-189.

Halmi, K. (1983). Anorexia Nervosa and Bulimia. *Psychosomatics, 24,* 111-129.

Halmi, K. (1982). Pragmatic information on eating disorders. *Psychiatric Clinics of North America, 52,* 371-377.

Halmi, K., Powers, P., & Cunningham, S. (1975). Treatment of Anorexia Nervosa with Behavior Modification. *Archives of General Psychiatry, 32,* 93-96.

Johnson, C., Lewis, C., & Hagman, J. (1984). The syndrome of bulimia, review and synthesis. *Psychiatric Clinics of North America, 7(2),* 247-273.

Turner, S., Calhoun, K., & Adams, H. (1981). *Handbook of Clinical Behavior Therapy.* New York: Wiley and Sons.

Ullmann, L. & Krasner, L. (1966). *Case Studies in Behavior Modification.* New York: Holt, Rinehart and Winston.

Vigersky, R. (Ed.). (1977). *Anorexia Nervosa.* New York: Raven Press.

Wolpe, J. (1969). *The Practice of Behavior Therapy.* New York: Pergamon Press.

Occupational Dysfunction and Eating Disorders: Theory and Approach to Treatment

Roann Barris, EdD, OTR

ABSTRACT. A review of literature on eating disorders in terms of the components of the model of human occupation suggests that eating disordered individuals are dysfunctional not only in their attitudes and habits related to eating and weight control, but also in their pursuit of and engagement in meaningful occupation. This article begins with a discussion of components of the model of human occupation and relevant research on eating disorders, using case vignettes to illustrate occupational dysfunction. The article concludes with the delineation of an occupational therapy approach to assessment and treatment of occupational dysfunction in eating disordered clients.

INTRODUCTION

Models for practice in occupational therapy should provide theoretical guidelines for working with general populations (Kielhofner & Barris, 1984). To be effective in terms of both generating research and influencing clinical practice, these models must clearly articulate their theoretical links with more global occupational therapy theory and knowledge, i.e., with the field's conceptual view of order, disorder, and approach to intervention or the restoration of order. The model of human occupation, originally proposed in 1980 and subsequently elaborated in other work, is a practice model

Roann Barris is Assistant Professor at University of Wisconsin-Madison, 1300 University Avenue, Madison, Wisconsin 53706.

This article is an expansion of the section on anorexia nervosa in the following chapter: Barris, R., Kielhofner, G., Neville, A., Oakley, F., Salz, C., & Watts, J. (in press). Psychosocial dysfunction. In Kielhofner, G. (Ed.), *The model of human occupation: Theory and application.* Baltimore: Williams & Wilkins.

27

which locates its theoretical origins in occupational behavior theory (Kielhofner & Burke, 1980; Kielhofner, 1980a; Kielhofner, 1980b; Kielhofner, Burke & Igi, 1980; Barris, 1983; Kielhofner & Burke, in press). This model is proving to be an effective means of examining physical and psychosocial disorders from a nonmedical perspective. In other words, the model allows occupational therapists to delineate problems related to occuaptional dysfunctions which may accompany, precede, or follow physical or emotional illnesses or trauma.

This article uses the model of human occupation as a framework for exploring the nature of occupational dysfunction that accompanies eating disorders and for delineating the contribution that occupational therapists can make to the remediation of these multifaceted disorders.

EATING DISORDERS

Because of the prevalence of eating disorders and the variation in their severity, several writers have suggested that a "continuum" of eating disorders may exist among young women (Garner, Olmsted, Polivy, & Garfinkel, 1984). In this continuum, anorexia nervosa, without the presence of bulimic symptoms (bingeing and purging) is placed at one extreme. Other eating disorders which are included in this spectrum are bulimia in conjunction with anorexia nervosa, bulimia as an entity in itself, weight-preoccupation in dieting women, and obesity. In some ways, bulimia has created the most difficulties for diagnosticians (despite the fact that it is now listed as a diagnostic entity in DSM-III) since there is evidence that the behaviors of bingeing and purging are very common among female college populations (Halmi, Falk, & Schwartz, 1981; Squire, 1983) thereby implying that these may actually be "normal" behaviors. In fact, recent research comparing weight-preoccupied women with anorexic women revealed that there were subgroups of weight-preoccupied women, with some exhibiting significant psychopathology and strongly resembling the anorexic and bulimic patients, while others were clearly closer in emotional well-being to women who were not weight-preoccupied (Garner et al., 1984). The issue therefore seems to be what distinguishes the maladaptive person who engages in severe dietary restriction or in bingeing and purging from the less maladaptive (Johnson, Lewis & Hagman, 1984).

Symptomatology and Etiology of Eating Disorders

Although most bulimic women weigh close to their normal body weight (Johnson et al.) both bulimia and anorexia have been characterized by an intense striving for thinness (Garner et al., 1984; Johnson et al., 1984). According to DSM-III (American Psychiatric Association, 1980), anorexia is further associated with a distorted body perception and a weight loss of approximately 25% of the original body weight. While no physical disease precipitates the disorder, the severe weight loss often leads to metabolic and other physical changes. These changes are usually responsible for bringing the individual to medical attention, since, as a rule, the person denies that anything is wrong and is resistive to treatment (American Psychiatric Association).

Anorexia nervosa generally afflicts female adolescents, many of whom come from middle- and upper-class families (Garner & Garfinkel, 1980; Jones, 1981). Anorexia has also been observed in women in young adulthood and is frequently a secondary diagnosis with another psychiatric disorder, e.g., depression or borderline personality disorder.

Bulimia has been distinguished from anorexia by its occurrence in women of near or normal weight. There is some evidence that bulimic women present at an older age (mid-twenties) after having symptoms for several years, and that a greater heterogeneity of socioeconomic status is represented in this group (Johnson et al.). Its identifying characteristics are binge-eating episodes followed by purging or restricting dietary intake. Typically, the binge is carried out in secrecy and consists of the rapid consumption of large amounts of carbohydrate foods in a fairly short period of time (American Psychiatric Association, 1980). However, recent studies describe much greater variation in the nature of the binge than is suggested by DSM-III and indicate that it is the experience or phenomenology of feeling out of control while eating, rather than the quantity of food consumed, that may determine whether a binge has occurred (Johnson et al., 1984).

Writers have typically focused on the family system as playing an important etiological role in anorexia, hypothesizing that these persons are overly dependent on their families and have difficulty developing autonomy while striving to meet parental expectations (Bruch, 1973; Moore & Coulman, 1981; Palazzoli, 1978). More recent formulations propose that an interaction of several factors contributes to the development of anorexia. These include a biological predisposition toward losing weight during periods of stress (more often a characteristic of females than males), a culture that values both thinness and achievement, and a lack of meaningful peer relationships (Jones, 1981). Both early and current perspectives recognize the struggle for identity and autonomy as key issues for the anorexic person.

The etiological model for bulimia is similar. Johnson et al. (1984) propose a biopsychosocial model in which the individual is first biologically at risk for the development of a major affective disorder. Second, the child grows up in a family environment with chaotic interpersonal relationships but a higher than average achievement orientation. This family environment is located within a sociocultural milieu that is also unstable in terms of the contradictory role expectations given to women. Finally, the young woman is also characterized by predisposing psychological factors such as high anxiety, impulsiveness, and low self-esteem. Ultimately, "the pursuit of thinness emerges as one very concrete activity in which young women can engage, that results in consistently favorable social responses that then enhance self esteem" (Johnson et al., p. 258).

EATING DISORDERS AND OCCUPATIONAL BEHAVIOR

As their name suggests, the behavior that stands out in these disorders concerns eating and attitudes toward food and weight. Nevertheless, certain distortions of occupational behavior also appear to be evident among these individuals. Reviewing existing literature in terms of the components of the model of human occupation allows a picture of the occupational dysfunction that accompanies eating disorders to emerge.

The model of human occupation is an open system view of the person which proposes that through ongoing interaction with the environment, the individual outputs various forms of occupation (i.e., work, play, and self-maintaining behaviors). The throughput stage of this model consists of three hierarchically arranged subsystems which motivate the person to interact with the environment and which produce and organize skilled behavior into meaningful patterns of habits and roles.

Volition

The volition subsystem is the highest subsystem in the hierarchy and represents the symbolic motivation to explore and master the environment. The components of this subsystem are personal causation, values, and interests. Personal causation refers to a view of oneself as effective, or as an origin in one's life (Burke, 1977), and reflects feelings of internal or external control (the belief that what happens is a result of either one's own actions or of external circumstances), feelings that one's actions are useful and efficacious, and expectations for success or failure in one's endeavors (Kielhofner & Burke, in press). Values, in the model of human occupation, refer to the meanings found in various occupations, to the standards of performance one holds, to goals for future occupations, and to one's orientation to past, present and future, and the meaning of this orientation in terms of occupational choices (Kielhofner & Burke, in press). Finally, interests are the tendencies or dispositions to find pleasure in certain occupations (Kielhofner & Burke; Matsutsuyu, 1969). Together, these components influence the decisions that one makes to engage in certain forms of occupation and the degree of challenge that one seeks in these occupations. Because volition is the highest level subsystem, it "governs" or influences the organization of the two lower subsystems.

Personal Causation and Eating Disorders

Locus of control appears to be a prominent issue among both bulimic and anorexic women. Traditionally, the anorexic female has been described as being involved in a struggle to attain internal control. Presumably, persons develop overly rigid eating patterns in response to feelings of helplessness (Bruch, 1970; Caspar & Davis, 1977). By reducing their food intake to the point of starvation, they strive to achieve a sense of control and feelings of worthiness from having done something "extraordinary" (Bruch, 1978).

Current research, however, is offering conflicting evidence to the assumption that anorexic persons are highly external. In fact, younger anorexic patients may score more internally than norms given for their age peers (Hood, Moore, & Garner, 1982). However, those anorexic patients who do score highly on external locus of control seem to be more apt to score highly on other measures of psychological disturbance (Hood et al.; Strober, 1982).

Bulimic women have also been characterized as having a strong need for control. As stated previously, the binge experience is one of extreme loss of control; for many, the following purge is a way of reasserting control (Johnson et al., 1984). One group of researchers has hypothesized that feelings of externality in bulimic women related in particular to sex-role behaviors (Rost, Neuhaus, & Florin, 1982)). This study found that although bulimic women did not differ markedly from their peers in terms of sex-role *attitudes,* the actual sex-role *behaviors* that they would endorse reflected a view that women were not truly in control of their lives.

Whatever their internal/external orientation, eating-disordered persons lack belief in the efficacy of their skills. For example, college women who admitted that they engaged in anorexic behaviors but were not acually diagnosed as having the illness all reported feelings of being inadequate to maintaining their own high standards or expectations (Squire, 1983).

An example of how extreme these feelings of inefficacy can be is found in the following client. Louise, a 17-year-old anorexic patient, had been hospitalized at least once a year for the previous five years. Louise had frequent mood swings, and depression was clearly interwoven with her anorexia. One assessment which she completed for the occupational therapists was a measure of automatic negative beliefs that a person might hold about him/herself (Hollon & Kendall, 1980). On this instrument, Louise scored well above the mean given for depressed patients, expressing an extreme lack of belief in herself and her abilities.

Values and Eating Disorders

The values of anorexic persons appear to be strongly shaped by the mass media and by their parents. By starving themselves, they carry the media image of the slender woman to its extremity (Rickarby, 1979). The anorexic teenager is also typically locked into her family system (Bruch, 1973; Moore & Coulman, 1981), and finds it difficult to resist the family's high valuation of achievement. Unfortunately, the goal of perfection which she sets for herself becomes entwined with her attempt to establish control over her body (Bruch, 1977).

Aimee Liu (Liu, 1979), a young woman who was anorectic from about the age of 12 until her college years, illustrates this interaction. When Aimee initially began dieting, it was in response to being slightly overweight for her age. After losing 15 pounds she felt that, for the first time, she had been in control of her life. Although Aimee was a top student, she felt that she was never as perfect as her parents and others expected her to be; losing more weight became her solution to the problem of perfection. As she became thinner, her dieting allowed her to achieve further independence in the form of job offers from modeling agencies. Of course, the modeling jobs only reinforced the notion that being thin was desirable.

The tendency to conform to social goals may also be manifested by conforming to subcultural group goals. Many of the anorexic-like women on college campuses are sorority members and influenced by these groups' strong emphasis on physical attractiveness (Squire, 1983). Anorexic and anorexic-type women are also over-represented among dance and modeling students (Garner & Garfinkel, 1980), two other subcultural groups that highly value thinness.

Although anorexic females are often perfectionists who set high standards of performance for themselves, their occupational goals are frequently unclear (Boskind-Lodahl, 1976; Squire). For both anorexic and bulimic young women there may also be a conflict between traditional feminine occupational values and changing cultural notions of feminine success (Boskind-Lodahl; Jones, 1981). Not knowing what their goals are or whether they can even attain them, they seize on the solution of changing their physique.

The meaning of activity and a feeling of purposefulness in life may also be distorted for eating disordered women. For example, many runners engage in this sport for the pleasure of it or as a way to cope with stress. For the anorexic person, however, physical activity may become primarily a means of controlling weight (Blumenthal, O'Toole, & Chang, 1984). Further, food-related activities may take the place of other activities and eventually be used to preclude feelings (Weinstein & Richman, 1984).

An overall sense of meaning in life may be diminished for bulimic women. In one sample of bulimic women, three-quarters expressed feelings of strong depersonalization (Abraham & Beaumont, 1982). Another case is illustrative. Penny was a 30-year-old woman who had never specifically sought help for her eating problems. Despite a reasonable level of achievement in her profession, she questioned the value of her work and had strong doubts about her future professional goals. On a multidimensional measure of life attitude (defined as the degree of existential meaning and purpose of life, and the motivation to find meaning and purpose) (Reker & Peacock, 1981), she scored substantially below age peers on life purpose, but higher than her age group on the will for meaning in life and goal-seeking. These discrepancies suggest a conflict arising from feelings of emptiness in her present daily life, combined with a strong drive for meaning oriented primarily toward the future.

Interests and Eating Disorders

Anorexic adolescents frequently have a wide range of interests, although athletic pursuits tend to be predominant (Gladston, 1974; Liu, 1979; MacLeod, 1981; Perkins, 1983). These adolescents are also often quite creative, but such interests may eventually become subordinate to preoccupations with dieting and exercise (Gladston). Despite avoidance of eating, food-related activities such as reading recipes and preparing gourmet meals for friends and family also may become dominant (Gladston; Larson & Johnson, 1981; Liu). The anorexic adolescent may also engage in far fewer social leisure activities than other adolescents (Jones, 1981; Larson & Johnson; Perkins). In the one empirical study of social and leisure adjustment of bulimic women, subjects were found to be significantly impaired, scoring similarly to a comparison group of alcoholic women (Johnson & Berndt, 1983). This study suggests that bulimic women share the social leisure deficiencies of anorexic women. In part this may be because preoccupations with food and food-related activities lead to diminished potency of former interests (Gladston; Johnson et al., 1984).

Habituation

Habituation is the middle level subsystem and is responsible for organizing behavior into routines. Its two components are habits and roles. A role is generally thought of as a collection of behaviors, attitudes, and status that accompanies a certain position in society (Black, 1976; Heard, 1977). Roles have occupational components if they serve to organize a person's use of time and involve some form of productive activities. The aspects of roles which are of concern in the model of human occupation are the person's perceptions of incumbency in a role (i.e., the person believes him/herself to occupy a particular role), the degree to which a person has internalized the behavioral and attitudinal expectations that accompany a role, and role balance, the ability to allot time to a variety of occupational roles (Kielhofner & Burke, in press). Habits are the other component of the habituation subsystem and are routine patterns of behavior that enable much of our daily occupational performance to be fairly automatic (Kielhofner, Barris, & Watts, 1982). To be adaptive, habits must be socially appropriate as well as relevant to a person's values, achieve a balance between too much flexibility and too much rigidity, and lead to effective management of time for work, play, self-care, and rest (Kielhofner & Burke, in press). The roles assumed by a person and the habits that accompany these roles are influenced by the volition subsystem and the person's motivation to engage in certain forms of occupational behavior. In turn, roles and habits influence the skills that a person will be motivated to develop.

Roles and Eating Disorders

The anorexic adolescent has strongly internalized the role of family member. The family unit of anorexic adolescents tends to be highly self-contained. Family members are often strongly invested in one another and struggle to keep conflict and differences beneath the surface. Because of this self-containment and over-investment, these families are somewhat isolated from the larger social structure (Jones, 1981).

Since the role of family member prevails in the life of the anorexic female, other roles may be less important or not as well internalized. The role of friend, for example, is often a marginal one for these adolescents (Jones; Larson & Johnson, 1981). In addition, although they have competently fulfilled the obligations of the student role, they often have difficulty making the transition into an adult worker role (Jones). For some anorexic adolescents, starvation may become a means of resolving the conflict between wanting to remain enmeshed in the family while realizing the need to prepare for a worker role (Jones). Certain occupational roles, however, may place the female at risk for developing anorexia. Occupations in which physique is pivotal, such as dancing, may have a larger than expected prevalence of anorexic members (Garner & Garfinkel, 1980).

Adrian, a young woman who had been anorexic for many years, exemplifies the over-internalization of the family role at the expense of other roles. Although Adrian was married and working, her primary adult work role was as a freelance artist. Interestingly, this work was carried out in collaboration with her father, despite the fact that working with him was stressful for her. Socially, she mentioned having several friends, but in actuality her primary social companion appeared to be her husband, whereas her other relationships remained superficial.

The bulimic woman may actually be more impaired in role performance than the anorexic woman. Partly because she is likely to be older, she may have taken on a worker role, although performance in this role may be impaired (Johnson & Berndt, 1983). Again, because of her age, she is less likely to be entrenched in her family; however, this may mean a greater likeliness of being isolated from others, particularly as her involvement with food starts to take precedence over involvement with family and friends (Johnson & Larson, 1982).

Many of the precipitating factors associated with the onset of bulimia concern role-related problems—work-related stress, family conflict, or loss of a social role (separation from friends, for example) (Johnson et al., 1984). In an interview concerning performance of the social leisure role (Good-Ellis, Fine & Spencer, 1984), Penny described a history of adequate social role performance throughout childhood and college. In her recent life, however, there was a paucity of social roles in her life. Because she had moved, the role of friend was not organizing her present life; in addition the role of family member was not a strong one for her. The worker role was currently her predominant role.

Habits and Eating Disorders

In many areas of her life, the anorexic person recognizes and conforms to socially expected habits. Academic habits, for example, are often highly effective. However, in the area of body weight, her habits are likely to be characterized by ritual and rigidity (Bruch, 1970; Jeanmet, 1981). Food rituals include not eating during family meals, playing with food on her plate so as to simulate eating, studying caloric values of food, preparing elaborate or gourmet dishes for others to consume, and secret bingeing. Weight-related rituals may consist of self-induced vomiting or the use of laxatives following the ingestion of food, and repeated weight checks to make sure she has not gained. The anorexic person often becomes excessively rigid in her food-related habits because of her fear of losing all control should she relax her vigil against weight gain (Bruch, 1970). This rigidity appears to be more characteristic of externally oriented anorexic persons than those who are more internal (Strober, 1982).

For the bulimic woman, eating rituals also become habitual. Because the binge-purge behavior is often secret, she may begin to spend increased amounts of time in private (Johnson & Larson, 1982). There is an interesting vicious cycle at play here: while the disordered eating behaviors may be partially a response to loneliness and isolation, they begin to necessitate a further increase in time spent alone. One survey of bulimic women found that respondents spent an average of 13.7 hours a week in bingeing and purging behaviors, most of this occurring in the evening (Johnson et al, 1984).

Performance

The performance subsystem is the lowest in the hierarchy and consists of perceptual-motor processes and interpersonal skills, and their neurologic, muscuoskeletal, and symbolic components (Kielhofner & Burke, in press). This subsystem enables action, and although it is governed by the two higher subsystems, it has the potential to constrain those two subsystems as well. In other words, if someone wants to be a surgeon, but lacks the fine motor and process skills that are necessary to that role, then successful performance is not likely to occur. However, the desire to achieve a certain goal may lead the person to strive to develop the essential skills.

Performance and Eating Disorders

Because the anorexic individual is often bright, creative and active, she superficially appears to have no skill deficits. In reality, however, she may have deficits in perceptual and interactional skills. First, the anorexic individual may misinterpret or incorrectly perceive bodily sensations, so that she denies feeling hunger or fatigue (Bruch, 1970), and after eating small amounts may feel unrealistically bloated. Perceptually, she does not recognize that she is emaciated and has an extremely distorted body image (Boskind-Lodahl, 1976; Bruch; Hood, Moore & Garner, 1982). Finally, anorexic persons often have poor social skills. Unlike "normal" individuals, they have few ties with peers, and the friendships that they do have tend to be short-lived (Jones, 1981).

Most bulimic women are college-educated, suggesting that cognitive process skills are not impaired. Little has been written about the perception of body image in bulimic subjects, although in normal weight subjects it is probably not likely to be impaired. Again, as with anorexic subjects, social skills may be deficient (Johnson & Berndt, 1983).

The Environment

In the model of human occupation, the person interacts with the external environment in an ongoing dynamic cycle. The environment, consisting of objects, tasks, social groups and organizations, and culture, can enhance or suppress the person's desire to explore and engage in his/her surroundings, and press for the development of certain behaviors and attitudes (Barris, 1983; Barris, Kielhofner, Levine, & Neville, in press). Through experience in an increasing variety of settings, the person becomes prepared to assume a variety of occupational roles (Barris, 1983). Thus, the human system/environment interaction can contribute to both the development and refinement of the internal components of the system as well as to the overall production of adaptive occupational behavior.

The Environment and Eating Disorders

Eating disorders seem to emerge in response to particular properties of the social and cultural environments. At the level of social groups, the family environment is pivotal for the anorexic adolescent. Because these families tend to have impermeable boundaries, risk taking and change are not encouraged, and the growing child does not playfully explore her surroundings or interact with peers. Hence, the environment is one which does not promote competence or a sense of mastery in the adolescent (Jones, 1981).

Further, the values of the family may conflict with cultural views. While her family tacitly does not encourage or expect independence, social norms do. The gap between family and societal values can be more easily breached when the adolescent has a strong peer network (Jones). The anorexic adolescent, however, is socially isolated, and finds it difficult to resolve the conflict productively (Jones).

The cultural environment is implicated in both anorexia and bulimia through the values it transmits about standards of feminine beauty (Jones) and which tend to recognize the worth of women for this physical attractiveness as opposed to their accomplishments (Boskind-Lodahl, 1976; Johnson et al., 1984). The young woman desiring recognition of her worth is torn between desiring recognition for achievement (the typically male avenue to external recognition) and finding that recognition is more readily available for physical beauty. Because her accomplishments may go unrecognized and unrewarded in a society that does not yet fully recognize and value accomplishment, the eating disordered woman may view control of her body through starvation or purging as a means of subverting this cultural norm (Boskind-Lodahl; Johnson et al.).

Eating disorders may also contribute to a gradual restriction of the environmental settings in which the person participates. For example, Penny, the bulimic subject described previously, had a routine which consisted of time spent at work, home, and the YMCA where she took an aerobics class a few nights a week. Only rarely did she engage in activities located in other settings. Similarly, Rosalyn, an anorexic patient in her mid-twenties, interacted in very few environments. On an inventory of important personally-chosen projects (Little, 1983), the location of six of ten projects listed was her home. One project was tied to the hospital and one to a dance school, and two projects had non-specific locations because they did not concern setting-specific behaviors (interacting with people and coping with certain types of stresses).

Summary: The Occupational Dynamic of Eating Disorders

Anorexics are frequently high competent and achieving persons, who, in effect, appear to have an almost exaggerated need for occupation. They are often involved in a tremendous amount of physical activity (Bruch, 1970), are very competitive, and excel in scholastic work (Garner & Garfinkel, 1980; Liu, 1979; MacLeod, 1981). However, apart from the physical exercise which is seen as a route to weight control, their conceptualization of the relationship between means and ends may be faulty (Strober, 1982). In other words the anorexic person may believe that by controlling her body weight, she will attain a sense of being an independent, competent person in all aspects of her life. Ironically, the effects of starvation may prevent her from successfully interacting with the environment.

The bulimic person may not always suffer from the same excessive need to be busy; however the meaning of occupation may be lost or subverted. As the eating-related activities become increasingly important, and other activities increasingly devoid of meaning, the bulimic person may find herself relying more and more on habit and routine to get through her days. Unfortunately, as her habits become rigid she locks herself more completely into a maladaptive occupational lifestyle.

OCCUPATIONAL THERAPY ASSESSMENT AND TREATMENT OF EATING DISORDERS

Therapists usually look for one assessment that can be used to provide a global picture of the client's functioning in a reasonably brief period of time. The assessments included here would probably require two or more hours to be administered. However, many of these instruments can be very self-revealing to the client; the therapist should consider that these assessments are actually the initiation of the treatment process.

The model of human occupation pinpoints several areas for assessment. The assessments to be described should provide detailed information on the status of model components.

Assessments

Reid-Ware Three-Factor Internal-External Scale (Reid & Ware, 1973; 1974)

This instrument is a paper-and-pencil measure of locus of control. It differs from earlier measures of locus in control in that it has been factor analyzed. As a result, the instrument yields three scores—a measure of fatalism, a measure of belief in control by social systems, and a measure of belief in self-control. The dimension of self-control probably is especially relevant to the eating disordered population.

Life Attitude Profile (Reker & Peacock, 1981)

Another paper-and-pencil instrument, the Life Attitude Profile provides information about the meaning and purpose of the person's daily life, the person's orientation to the future, and the person's will to find meaning in life. This instrument may be useful to confirm the degree to which meaninglessness is present in the bulimic individual's current lifestyle.

Leisure and Work History

While a lack of interests does not appear to be a problem for eating disordered women, the reasons for engaging in interests and the satisfactions obtained from them may be. A semi-structured interview exploring the subjects's history of involvement in leisure and work could be used to identify such themes as: the extent to which past and present activities are solitary or social; reasons typically given for taking up or dropping activities; playfulness experienced during activities; the degree of competence experienced during activities, and other trends. For the older subject, especially the bulimic woman, work satisfaction may be a particularly important area for focus. Some supplementary paper-and-pencil measures that could also be used include the Leisure Satisfaction Scale (Beard & Ragheb, 1980) which examines a variety of reasons for engaging in leisure and the WHY Scale (Day, 1979), a measure of the degree to which extrinsic and intrinsic factors are involved in a person's motivation for particular activities.

The Role Checklist (Oakley, Kielhofner & Barris, 1984; Barris, Oakley & Kielhofner, in press).

This is a quick screening instrument that examines the person's perceptions of incumbency in ten roles in the past and present, and intent to assume these roles in the future. The instrument also asks about the degree of value given to each role. With the eating disordered client, this instrument may provide a graphic indication of the extent to which roles are or are not available to structure the person's life.

The Role Performance Scale
(Good-Ellis, Fine, & Spence, 1984)

This instrument uses an interview format and a rating scale that is applied to the resulting data. Parallel interviews have been developed for 12 roles; each yields a picture of past performance in that role as well as performance in a particular time interval prior to administration. The instrument thus enables identification of changes in role performance, factors that influenced changes, and how stressful events have affected role performance. Since role performance can be a critical problem area for eating disordered clients, this instrument may be especially useful.

Occupational Questionnaire
(Riopel, 1982)

Time use is another extremely critical area. The Occupational Questionnaire is an activities configuration which asks the individual to provide detailed information on time use and to rate activities carried out in terms of their meaningfulness (importance), pleasure, and competence felt during the activity. The instrument therefore yields information on habits, rigidity of time use, and personal reactions to how time is used.

Projects Inventory
(Little, 1983)

This is not a formal assessment but an approach to examining the personal projects of importance in an individual's life. This format may be useful to identify conflicts between values and chosen projects, degree of satisfaction in projects, external supports and constraints for project completion, and finally, the environmental location of projects.

Treatment

Therapeutic approaches used by other mental health professionals have tended to focus on identification of faulty cognitive beliefs (e.g., the need to be excessively thin), the underlying psychodynamics of the eating disorder, and direct change through behavioral interventions of the eating habits (Fairburn, 1981; Lacey, 1983; Johnson et al., 1984; Weinstein & Richman, 1984; Bruch, 1970). While these are all valid areas of concern, they seem to skirt the possibility that other activities, apart from eating, may also be disordered. The occupational therapist can contribute to the multidisciplinary care of the eating disordered individual by focusing on dysfunction in occupational behavior.

For example, the eating disordered person needs to increase her feeling of comfort in situations requiring risk taking and flexibility without the necessity of achieving; play is an essential medium for accomplishing this. In addition, she must begin to visualize herself as moving into an independent adult worker role. To this end, the pleasurable experience of both work and leisure occupations is necessary, so that she can perceive herself as efficacious and capable of entering the occupational choice process.

The development of more extensive peer networks is another area for occupational therapy intervention. Situations in which the eating-disordered person can enact the friendship role should be identified and incorporated into the therapeutic process. For instance, the client can be encouraged to find ways of enacting existing hobbies within an organizational context, such as joining an orchestra, taking a continuing education course, or folk dancing.

Increasing awareness of the reasons for engaging in activities and the satisfactions found in them might be accomplished by keeping a journal. Writing may also come to be seen as a pleasing activity that the client can turn to during periods of emptiness. Values clarification activities may be useful to this end as well.

The eating disordered person should be encouraged to experiment with changing routines and new activities to decrease the feelings of being out of control that may accompany change. By deliberately planning a different schedule for certain days of the week, the client can still feel in control of life without being rigid. Choosing a new activity or event to try out on a weekly basis will also bring the client into contact with new environments and social groups.

These suggestions are just a framework for a therapeutic program with eating disordered individuals. Obviously, the seriousness of the disorder, whether or not the client is hospitalized, the client's age, and other factors will all affect treatment decisions. Ultimately, for the eating disordered client, the focus of occupational therapy intervention should be on enabling the person to feel in control of and satisfied with her participation in meaningful occupations.

REFERENCES

Abraham, S.F., & Beumont, P.J.V. (1982). How patients describe bulimia or binge eating. *Psychological Medicine, 12,* 625-635.

American Psychiatric Association. (1980). *Diagnostic and statistical manual of mental disorder,* 3rd edition. Washington, D.C.: American Psychiatric Association.

Barris, R. (1983). Environmental interactions: An extension of the model of human occupation. *American Journal of Occupational Therapy, 36,* 627-644.

Barris, R., Kielhofner, G., Levine, R., & Neville, A. (in press). Occupation as interaction with the environment. In Kielhofner, G. (Ed.), *The model of human occupation: Theory and application*. Baltimore: Williams & Wilkins.

Barris, R., Oakley, F., & Kielhofner, G. (in press). The role checklist. In Hemphill, B. (Ed.), *The evaluative process in psychiatric occupational therapy*, 2nd edition. Thorofare, NJ: Slack.

Beard, J.G., & Ragheb, M.G. (1980). Measuring leisure satisfaction. *Journal of Leisure Research, 12*, 20-33.

Black, M. (1976). The occupational career. *American Journal of Occupational Therapy, 30*, 225-228.

Blumenthal, J.A., O'Toole, L.C., & Chang, J.L. (1984). Is running an analogue of anorexia nervosa? *Journal of the American Medical Association, 252*, 520-523.

Boskind-Lodahl, M. (1976). Cinderella's stepsisters: A feminist perspective on anorexia nervosa and bulimia. *Journal of Women in Culture and Society, 2*, 342-356.

Bruch, H. (1970). Changing approaches to anorexia nervosa. *International Psychiatric Clinics, 7*, 3-24.

Bruch, H. (1973). *Eating disorders*. NY: Basic.

Bruch, H. (1977). Psychological antecedents of anorexia nervosa. In Vigersky, R.A. (Ed.), *Anorexia nervosa*. NY: Raven.

Burke, J. (1977). A clinical perspective on motivation: Pawn versus origin. *American Journal of Occupational Therapy, 31*, 254-258.

Casper, R.C., & Davis, J.M. (1977). On the course of anorexia nervosa. *American Journal of Psychiatry, 131*, 974-978.

Day, H.I. (1979). Why people play. *Losir et Societe, 2*, 129-147.

Fairburn, C. (1981). A cognitive behavioral approach to the treatment of bulimia. *Psychological Medicine, 11*, 707-711.

Garner, D.M., Olmsted, M.P., Polivy, J., & Garfinkel, P.E. (1984). Comparison between weight-preoccupied women and anorexia nervosa. *Psychosomatic Medicine, 46*, 255-266.

Garner, D.N. & Garfinkel, P.E. (1980). Socio-cultural factors in the development of anorexia nervosa. *Psychological Medicine, 10*, 647-656.

Gladston, R. (1974). Mind over matter: Observations on 50 patients hospitalized with anorexia nervosa. *Journal of the American Academy of Child Psychiatry, 13*, 246-263.

Good-Ellis, M., Fine, S.B., & Spencer, J.H., Jr. (1984). The Role Performance Scale. Unpublished instrument, available from Payne-Whitney Psychiatric Clinic, 525 E. 68th St., NYC, NY.

Heard, G. (1977). Occupational role acquisition: A perspective on the chronically disabled. *American Journal of Occupational Therapy, 31*, 243-247.

Hollon, S.D., & Kendall, P.C. (1980). Cognitive self-statements in depression: Development of an automatic thoughts questionnaire. *Cognitive Therapy and Research, 4*, 383-398.

Hood, J., Moore, T.E., & Garner, B.M. (1982). Locus of control as a measure of ineffectiveness in anorexia nervosa. *Journal of Consulting and Clinical Psychology. 50*, 3-13.

Jeanmet, P. (1981). The anorectic stance. *Journal of Adolescence, 4*, 113-129.

Johnson, C., & Berndt, D.J. (1983). Preliminary investigation of bulimia and life adjustment. *American Journal of Psychiatry, 140*, 774-777.

Johnson, C., & Larson, R. (1982). Bulimia: An analysis of moods and behavior. *Psychosomatic Medicine, 44*, 341-351.

Johnson, C., Lewis, C., & Hagman, J. (1984). The syndrome of bulimia: Review and synthesis. *Psychiatric Clinics of North America, 7*, 247-273.

Jones, D. (1981). Structural discontinuity and the development of anorexia nervosa. *Sociological Focus, 3*, 233-247.

Kielhofner, G. (1980a). A model of human occupation, Part II. *American Journal of Occupational Therapy, 34*, 657-663.

Kielhofner, G. (1980b). A model of human occupation, Part III. *American Journal of Occupational Therapy, 34,* 777-778.

Kielhofner, G., & Barris, R. (1984). The organization of knowledge in occupational therapy. Submitted for publication.

Kielhofner, G., & Burke, J. (1980). A model of human occupation, Part I. *American Journal of Occupational Therapy, 34,* 572-581.

Kielhofner, G., & Burke, J. (in press). Components and determinants of human occupation. In Kielhofner, G. (Ed.), *The model of human occupation: Theory and application.* Baltimore: Williams & Wilkins.

Kielhofner, G., Barris, R., & Watts, J. (1982). Habits and habit dysfunction: A clinical perspective for psychosocial occupational therapy. *Occupational Therapy in Mental Health, 2,* 1-22.

Lacey, H.H. (1983). Bulimia nervosa, binge eating, and psychogenic vomiting: A controlled treatment study and long term outcome. *British Medical Journal, 286,* 1609-1613.

Larson, R., & Johnson, C. (1981). Anorexia nervosa in the context of daily experience. *Journal of Youth and Adolescence, 10,* 455-471.

Little, B.R. (1983). Personal projects: A rationale and method for investigation. *Environment and Behavior, 15,* 273-309.

Liu, A. (1979). *Solitaire: A narrative.* NY: Harper & Row.

MacLeod, S. (1981). *The art of starvation.* London: Virago.

Matsutsuyu, J.S. (1969). The interest checklist. *American Journal of Occupational Therapy, 23,* 323-328.

Moore, J.H., & Coulman, R.N. (1981). Anorexia nervosa: The patient, her family and key family therapy interventions. *Journal of Psychiatric Nursing and Mental Health Services, 19,* 9-14.

Oakley, F., Kielhofner, G., & Barris, R. (1984). The role checklist. Submitted for publication.

Palazzoli, M.S. (1978). *Self-starvation.* NY: Jason Aronson.

Perkins, E. (1983). The patterns, meanings, and need-satisfaction of leisure activities for eating disordered and non-eating disordered female adolescents. Unpublished master's project, Virginia Commonwealth University, Richmond, VA.

Reid, D.W., & Ware, E.E. (1974). Multidimensionality of internal versus external control: Addition of a third dimension and non-distinction of self versus others. *Canadian Journal of Behavioral Science, 6,* 132-142.

Reid, D.W., & Ware, E.E. (1973). Multidimensionality of internal-external control: Implications for past and future research. *Canadian Journal of Behavioral Science, 5,* 264-271.

Reker, G.T., & Peacock, E.J. (1981). The life attitude profile: A multidimensional instrument for assessing attitudes toward life. *Canadian Journal of Behavioural Science, 13,* 264-273.

Rickarby, G.A. (1979). Psychological dynamics in anorexia nervosa. *Medical Journal of Australia, 1,* 587-589.

Riopel, N.J. (1982). An examination of the occupational behavior and life satisfaction of the elderly. Unpublished master's project, Virginia Commonwealth University, Richmond, VA.

Rost, W., Neuhaus, M., & Florin, I. (1982). Bulimia nervosa: Sex role attitude, sex role behavior, and sex role related locus of control in bulimariexic women. *Journal of Psychosomatic Research, 26,* 403-408.

Squire, S. (1983). Is the binge-purge cycle catching? *Ms Magazine,* October, pp. 41-42, p. 46.

Strober, M. (1982). Locus of control, psychopathology, and weight gain in juvenile anorexia nervosa. *Journal of Abnormal Child Psychopathology, 10,* 97-106.

Weinstein, H.M., & Richman, A. (1984). The group treatment of bulimia. *Journal of American College Health, 32,* 208-215.

Occupational Therapy in the Rehabilitation of the Patient with Anorexia Nervosa

Gordon Muir Giles, BA, DIP COT
Mary Elizabeth Allen, MS, OTR

ABSTRACT. The first part of this paper develops an ecological and rehabilitative stance for the occupational therapist in relation to the anorexic patient. Maximizing the individual's level of psychosocial functioning is regarded as the primary aim of treatment. A model for approaching the anorexic patient is described which examines environmental factors, and the importance of assessment and follow up. The cognitive behavioral approach is discussed and suggestions are made for adapting it to the occupational therapist's orientation towards practical activity. In the second part of the paper concrete suggestions for therapy are made.

INTRODUCTION

It is difficult to assess the exact prevalence of anorexia nervosa as individuals with the disorder are frequently reluctant to seek help. The reported incidence of the disorder has however increased rapidly over the last 20 years so that it is now recognized as a relatively common condition.[1] Current estimates vary between 0.23[2] and 1.6[3] new cases annually per 100,000 population. Women make up the vast majority of sufferers, with men comprising only 5-10% of the total. Despite the prevalence of anorexia nervosa it has received lit-

Mary Elizabeth Allen, M.S., O.T.R., is Assistant Director at the Occupational Therapy Department, University of Wisconsin Hospital. Gordon Muir Giles is an Occupational Therapist at St. Andrews Hospital, Kensley Unit, Occupational Therapy Department, Northampton NNI 5DG England.

The authors wish to thank Elisabeth Cracknell, Director of the School of Occupational Therapy, Northampton, and to Dr. Peter Eames, Consultant Neuropsychiatrist, Jo Clark-Wilson Occupational Therapist, and Gill Shaw, all of The Kemsley Unit, St. Andrews Hospital, Northampton, for commenting on earlier drafts of this paper. Any error of fact or interpretation is, however, the sole responsibility of the authors.

tle attention in the occupational therapy literature.[4] In a sense this lack of written material has been a reflection of the state of treatment. It is only over the last 5-10 years that formal treatment programs for eating disorders have been developed. Prior to this the anorexic patient was either hospitalized on a medical unit and seen individually by a psychiatrist, or treated among the general psychiatric population.[5] In the former case the anorexic patient was often not referred to occupational therapy at all or at best referred for strengthening exercises just prior to discharge. Occasionally referrals were made to "give them something to do". When trying to develop a treatment program in a psychiatric unit the occupational therapist would have to treat the anorexic among seriously disturbed and psychotic patients and was therefore often unable to meet the needs of the anorexic patient. However, with the advent of eating disorders units (EDU) the occupational therapist has been able to develop specialized treatment programs to meet the complex demands of this patient population.

CURRENT LITERATURE

There is very little published material about the work of the occupational therapist with the anorexic patient. The majority of work that relates to occupational therapy has to do with body image distortions or follow-up studies of multidisciplinary treatment approaches and a number of these are briefly reviewed in this section. Since there are usually only one or two relevant studies in other areas discussion of these is reserved to treatment sections in the text.

A comprehensive review of the literature revealed only two papers specifically addressing occupational therapy with anorexic patients. The first is that by Martin[5] which is focused primarily on the occupational therapists use of art. Further discussion of this paper will occur in the section on art therapy. The second article is that of Giles and Chng which focuses on the use of a contractual-coping approach in the treatment of anorexia nervosa. Giles and Chng regard the negotiation of a contract as helpful in establishing a basis for treatment and in helping the patient to keep constantly in mind her own individual aims.[6] To be effective, the contract should be specific to the needs of the patient. The contract makes clear that the patient herself is responsible for change and that her success will often depend on her degree of motivation. A contract also reminds the therapist of the importance of initial and continuing assessment.

A number of authors have described the use of social skills training with this client population. The psychodynamic model of Bruch[7,8] and others sees the anorexic individual as feeling overwhelmed and smothered by others. One of the most consistent findings from follow up studies on anorexia nervosa are the social anxiety and isolation of patients. However, despite the apparent theoretical justification for SST with these patients, little research has actually been done into its efficacy. Most studies are limited to the single case study design which, though valid in itself, cannot substitute for controlled trials.[9,10] The only controlled trial known to the present authors is that by Pillay and Crisp[11] into the impact of SST with an established in-patient treatment program for anorexia nervosa. Unfortunately this study is so beset by methodological problems that it is impossible to draw any firm conclusions from it. In the view of the present authors SST and art therapy are currently justified on theoretical and practical grounds, though clearly research is needed in this area.

Body image distortion is a major area of discussion in the literature. Results of studies evaluating the perceptual component of the body image of patients with anorexia nervosa have been inconsistent. Fries[12] found that body perception indices significantly differentiated his anorexic subjects from controls, a finding which agreed with the previous results of Slade and Russell.[13] However, since several controls overestimated their size by 21% to 33% Fries was not convinced that overestimation was specific to anorexia nervosa. Button et al.,[14] found no significant differences between anorexic subjects and controls, both of whom overestimated body size. Marked overestimation by anorexics was however associated with an early relapse. In contrast to the Button study, results by Wingate and Christie[15] showed significant differences between controls and anorexic patients in the perception of body width when the mean age of subjects and controls was identical. Such a finding is contrary to the notion that age differences may explain observed perceptual differences between anorexics and controls which had been a criticism of earlier studies.

Garfinkel et al.[16] investigated the clinical outcome of anorexics in terms of their self-perception of body size. Those patients with poor outcomes were overestimators. Those with excellent outcomes were underestimators. They suggested treatment be directed towards improving self-perception if patients benefited only marginally from conventional therapy.

From the above research results as well as from recent reviews the most appropriate summary statements that can be derived regarding macrosomatognosia and anorexia nervosa are that (1) overestimation of body width is not unique to patients with a diagnosis of anorexia nervosa and (2) overestimation is associated with an unfavorable clinical outcome for anorexic patients.[4] Part of the current disagreement may be explained by the fact that the term "body image distortion" is ambiguous. The tendency for the anorexic patient to view herself as fat when clearly emaciated may reflect a labeling process rather than an actual perceptual distortion. The "distortion" may in fact be the result of a learned reaction to the appearance of thinness. Clearly, however, the fact that statements about perceived body size can be a prognostic indicator show that further study may be useful.

The last few years have brought relatively little clear progress in the treatment of anorexia nervosa.[1] It is still not known whether any form of treatment has any real effect on the natural history of the disorder. Morgan and Russell[17] show typical findings in their study of 41 inpatients, follow up was between four and ten years after discharge from hospital. In measures based on weight and menstrual function, 39 per cent were rated as showing "good", 27 per cent "intermediate", and 29 per cent "poor" outcome. Two of the patients, five per cent of the total, had died. In another study using comparable criteria, Hsu et al.,[18] found amongst their 49 inpatients 45 per cent "good", 37 per cent "intermediate", and 16 per cent "poor" outcome with one death (2 per cent). Most of the subjects in both studies retained a marked concern about their shape and weight, and other psychiatric symptoms were not uncommon. A third study using compatible criteria but on an out-patient group has recently been reported by Morgan et al.[19] with largely similar results. The subject's ability to work was usually unaffected, but many continued to have problems in forming close relationships, and were socially isolated. These results justify the occupational therapist's current orientation towards this patient group in concentrating on directly food-related problems and psychosocial functioning rather than work related areas.

Only one recent outcome study has included a discussion of occupational therapy in any depth. Although the results of this study were encouraging[20] it is not possible to assess the effect of the occupational therapy input because of the many treatment approaches used. We can currently base our intervention strategies only on evidence which seems suggestive of good outcome from other sources, and on the generalization of approaches which have been used effectively elsewhere.

THE TEAM APPROACH

The occupational therapist works in close co-operation with other members of the treatment team and can add her expertise in assessment and treatment planning as well as the practice of realistic life skills. An effective treatment team requires the participation of a consultant psychiatrist, clinical psychologist, physician, dietician, occupational therapist, social worker, and nursing staff. One appropriately qualified member of the treatment team should be designated as psychotherapist for each patient.

With the current emphasis on in-patient care, treatment of the anorexic patient will usually fall into two phases. Initially the medical intervention is primary and is directed towards stabilizing the patient's physical condition and helping her work through her acute psychological reaction to weight gain. The second part of treatment will involve an attempt to help the patient stabilize her weight and work on her problems through some form of psychotherapy. It is in this later stage that the rehabilitative approach of the occupational therapist is most useful.

The overall treatment approach on any individual EDU or other treatment setting is likely to reflect prevailing theories of causation. Current treatment approaches include the medical,[21] psychoanalytic,[22] family therapy,[23] behavioral[24] and more recently the cognitive behavioral approaches.[25] These approaches have been more fully described elsewhere.[26] The type of treatment approach used will also effect the likelihood, length, and quality of hospitalization.

In our view both occupational therapists and other professionals have underestimated the possible role of occupational therapy in the treatment of the anorexic patient. The occupational therapist is an expert in rehabilitation with a special emphasis on functional ability. The aim of the occupational therapist with this population, as with any other, should be to help the patient achieve the highest attainable level of psychological, physical and social competence. We will argue below that this rehabilitative approach is the one best suited to the needs of the anorexic patient.

THE REHABILITATIVE AND ECOLOGICAL MODELS

Although in general terms a number of factors are clearly implicated in the cause of anorexia nervosa, the actual causes in any individual case often remain obscure. What is clear is that once the condition is established a vast array of secondary factors can operate to maintain the abnormal pattern of eating behavior.

Figure 1 makes this point diagrammatically. Primary factors are those factors which in any particular causative theory are presumed

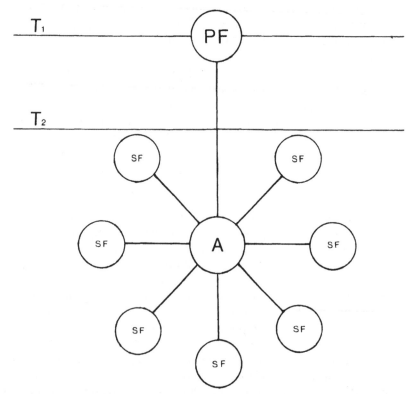

FIGURE 1. The Ecological Model. PF = Primary Factors. SF = Secondary factors. A = The Anorexic Patient. T1 = Time at Onset. T2 = Current State.

to be pathognomonic of the disorder. Secondary factors are those factors which, although not originally implicated in cause, support the continuation of the condition once established. For example, according to the psychodynamic theories of Bruch[7] primary factors might include low feelings of self efficacy, low self esteem and perfectionistic tendencies. Advocates of other causative models would cite other variables: e.g., the family interaction school would cite abnormal family dynamics as a major causative factor.[23]

Secondary factors might include things such as enjoying the sense of mastery associated with the control over eating,[8] avoiding the effects of sexual maturation, and gaining the admiration—albeit ambivalent—of peers.[27] Perhaps of more importance is the anorexic individual's changing reactions to food and eating arising as a consequence of the initial dieting behavior. These factors might include the effects of classical conditioning,[28] differentiation of the inner states of hunger and satiety,[29] and the tendency to binge which may be present in almost all "restrained" eaters.[30] Others have suggested that the anorexic's endogenous opioid system may act as a potent internal reinforcement for her dieting behavior.[31] Pickar et al.[32] found raised level of opioid activity in patients with anorexia nervosa during periods of minimum weight. Restoration of body weight was associated with decreases in opioid activity. The cause of the raised levels of opioid activity is not known but is consistent with the growing evidence linking the endogenous opioid system to stress reponse and the growing speculation about the link between these substances and the experience of pleasure.[33] Slade[34] has discussed the maintenance of the anorexic's abnormal eating patterns in behavioral terms. He suggested that the dieting behavior once begun is reinforced positively by the resulting feelings of success and satisfaction, and negatively through the fear of weight gain and the avoidance of other problems.

As occupational therapists our approach should be ecological, in that we emphasize current state and look at the patient's interaction with her environment. Since there may be not only a unique constellation of causative factors but an even more complex system of factors serving to maintain the condition, it seems reasonable to gear our treatment specifically to the needs of the individual sufferer. As long as our knowledge of the etiology of the disorder remains incomplete, our therapeutic interventions are likely to remain symptomatic.

In working with the anorexic patient the basic aims of treatment must be: (1) restoration of a healthy body weight and adequate eating habits and (2) psychological adjustment involving reduction of weight phobia. The goal of treatment is not "cure" but the achievement of the maximum level of psychosocial functioning possible for the individual concerned.

TREATMENT PLANNING

The first step in treatment is assessment. All relevant factors need to be included if an assessment is to be effective. Biological, social and psychological factors must all be considered. The purpose of the assessment is to identify the problems and by carefully examining them to come up with an effective strategy for dealing with them. Kanfer and Saslow[35] recommend viewing behavior in terms of: (1) behavioral excesses, (2) behavioral deficits and (3) behavioral assets. It is important for the occupational therapist to look for strengths as well as deficits because the former can often be used to overcome the latter.

The initial assessment is conducted using an interview format. It addresses the following major areas: activities of daily living (personal; PADL and domestic; DADL), social skills, cognitive deficits, work, and leisure pursuits. The patient is interviewed during the initial visit to the occupational therapy department. The therapist may also interview the patients family and/or friends as appropriate.

The PADL assesses hygiene, dressing, feeding and presentation skills. Is the patient well groomed? Is bathing timely and adequate? Does the patient dress appropriately for temperature and occasion. Do clothes fit appropriately? Is patient able to select foods appropriately and feed herself in functional manner without obsessional characteristics? Does patient interact with others during meal times?

The DADL assess domestic activities of daily living which included ability to do household task such as washing clothes, vacuuming, dusting. In addition budgeting, meal planning, shopping for both food and clothes, particular attention should be paid to food preparation and storage.

Social skills including ability to form and maintain meaningful social relationships is also investigated in the initial interview. Note is made of the patients ability to be assertive in making her wants known.

Cognitive deficits particularly attention and concentration are assessed. Focus is on the patient's ability to make reasoned judgments both outside and within the areas of overvalued ideas. It is important to look at this area in terms of the patient's ability to be functional even though she may have some faulty or obsessional thinking.

Another major area to be assessed by the therapist is that of work/school. Although this area is not typically a problem it is still necessary to confirm that the patient is functional in these areas. As these patients are more usually high/overachievers work and school performance ratings are quite good. It just may be this level of high intensity that creates a balance problem. Is the patient putting all her time and energy into this performance area and not meeting her other needs in the areas of self care and leisure?

Leisure pursuits and hobbies are ascertained through the use of an interest inventory initially filled out by the patient and then further discussed in a follow-up session to ascertain the significance of the pursuits chosen.

Notation is also made of the patients admitting physical examination report from the medical record as well as the results of the routine stress test indicating blood pressure, general cardiac history and status. A quick assessment is also made of the patient's general endurance and abdominal strength as these are frequent problem areas.

After the initial interview practical assessments of such things as, shopping, cooking, and feeding, are de rigeur. The therapist can also assess any other problem areas which may have been suggested by the initial interview.

Once assessment is completed and the areas of deficit are isolated, performance can be practiced. Learning can be seen to have taken place through a decreasing variability in performance and an increasing smoothness and accuracy in execution. Once performance is adequate it can be integrated into the patient's everyday activities. Initially follow-up should be regular; this can be gradually curtailed though the patient should understand that the occupational therapist is ready to assist should problems arise. The course of treatment can therefore be summarized as:

1. Assessment
2. Practice (areas of deficit)
3. Integration
4. Follow-up

The approach of the occupational therapist to the problems of the anorexic patient is activity oriented.[26] The patient is never a passive recipient of treatment, as she may be initially on the ward. So for example if a patient shows extreme anxiety about eating and weight gain, rather than placing the patient under pressure to conform a problem solving approach may be found more useful. The patient is encouraged to use coping techniques which she has been taught in occupational therapy such as anxiety reducing activities (yoga, relaxation, or preferred diversional activities) or by examining her own inappropriate thoughts and catastrophic expectations.

THE COGNITIVE BEHAVIORAL APPROACH

The tendency to choose either a psychotherapeutic or a behavioral approach leads to a failure to recognize the link between cognitive and behavioral factors: those approaches which exclusively address either cognition or behavior are likely to prove ineffective as a result. Let us take psychotherapy as an example: most authorities on the subject of eating disorders regard some form of psychoytherapy as an essential part of treatment.[1,7,23,25] However, a psychodynamic approach used in isolation from other intervention strategies may not enable the patient to overcome all her practical difficulties. It is one thing for the patient to gain insight into her eating pattern through psychotherapy, and quite another for her to behave approporiately when faced with the task of preparing food for herself or others. We will briefly examine the cognitive behavioral approach to see how this can be used by the occupational therapist.

Cognitive therapy emphasizes the role of negative cognitive distortion in many forms of mental disorder. Although it was originally designed by Beck and his co-workers[36] for use with depressive, neurotic and obsessive-compulsive subjects, many now consider cognitive therapy appropriate in the treatment of anorexia nervosa and bulimia.[25,37]

Faulty constructions of reality are considered to have detrimental effect on the individual's behavior and emotions. Although the patient's behavior appears illogical, it may be quite logically based on certain fundamental premises and beliefs about thinness and weight loss. The main form of therapy is therefore the examination of the patient's thoughts and ideas about herself in relation to food and eating. Within cognitive therapy certain therapeutic techniques are designed to identify, test, and correct distorted conceptualizations.

These techniques include Prospective Hypothesis-Testing, "what if" techniques, and decentering; these are described fully elsewhere.[25,36] The individual is taught to monitor negative automatic thoughts and to recognize the connection between cognition and behavior. The patient is encouraged to examine evidence for and against "automatic thoughts", e.g., "this food is bad and instantly converted to fat", and can be taught to identify and replace beliefs which lead to inappropriate behavior.

Despite the many advantages of a cognitive behavioral approach, practical activity has been inadequately stressed. Particular negative thoughts will arise and be dealt with more spontaneously in the relevant situations e.g., helping a patient work through her inappropriate thoughts about cooking and eating a meal would be most effectively done while cooking and eating. Once the area of difficulty is isolated the patient must practice alternative ways of behaving. Once this link has been made cognitive therapy becomes well suited to the functional problem-solving skills of the occupational therapist.

For example, Joan, an 18 year old with a two year history of anorexia, was being seen as an out patient in the eating disorders clinic. During the initial occupational therapy cooking assessment it was discovered that she would only allow herself to eat between the hours of midnight and 3:30 a.m. She explained this by stating her belief that eating at other times would lead her to binge and to become overweight. The therapists' approach to this problem was to explore with a patient the likely truth values of these thoughts. The patient was encouraged to consider the likely effect of expanding the period of time during which she allowed herself to eat by one half hour. The patient was able to acknowledge that her catastrophic expectations were erroneous and was gradually able to resume a more normal eating schedule.

THERAPEUTIC ACTIVITIES

No activity is in itself therapeutic for the anorexic patient. For an activity to become therapeutic it is important for both the therpist and the patient tò be committed to designing activities which will help the patient change. In order to do this the patient and therapist should try to establish concrete goals for each session. Before the patient can decide how she wants to change she needs first to find out about herself as she currently is. This idea of self discovery may also be set up in the form of a contract.

The therapeutic activities used by the occupational therapist can be classed as either functional approaches or expressive techniques. Under functional approaches can be grouped those activities where the emphasis is clearly on the practice of skills for independent living or the overcoming of physical deficits. Here examples might include cooking and clothes shopping. These activities can also be used to help the patient produce adaptive cognitive and behavioral change. Under expressive techniques are grouped those activities which are not directly relevant to the individual's normal life outside the treatment setting but are used because of their ability to provoke adaptive changes in the way the patient interacts with and thinks about her environment and herself. Examples of this second type of activity are movement and expressive art groups. Below is a description of various therapeutic activities which can be used in the treatment of the anorexic patient.

FUNCTIONAL APPROACHES

Cooking Assessment and Practice

Clearly central to the anorexic individual's problems are her inappropriate behavior around food and her reluctance to eat. The patient's preoccupation with calorie content often prevents her from being able to produce a well-balanced, "ordinary" meal. Meals should include normal "non-anorexic" foods and should not revolve around food fads.[38]

In the later stages of treatment when the patient may be shopping for herself, the occupational therapist should determine if the patient can prepare a shopping list, estimate quantities of food to be purchased, cook what is generally regarded as a nutritionally balanced meal, and dispose of unused food and waste correctly (i.e., without bingeing). The occupational therapist should be present during the shopping, cooking and eating of the meal. She can provide moral support and, where necessary, can prompt the use of coping techniques to resolve conflicts precipitated by the cooking practice. Initially when Pam was sent to the store to get food for a meal she would frequently spend large sums on her favored "junk food" and binge on it immediately after leaving the store. It took frequent practice with the occupational therapist before Pam could successfully shop. From a cognitive standpoint the opportunity of cooking practice can be used to examine faulty information-processing and thinking "styles".

Holmgrens et al.,[20] describe a program run by the occupational therapist at Uppsala University Hospital in Sweden. Initially patients prepare their own meals starting with exact amounts of basic ingredients. Later the patient is expected to plan her meal, shop and cook for herself. Later still the patient will be expected to cook for a group and to help herself to food without calculating the exact amount. Previously "forbidden" foods, the consumption of which in the past would have inevitably led to a binge, are also included in this later phase. Snack foods eaten with coffee in the cafeteria are included in the program. This is done to make the subsequent eating of such foods less catastrophic for the patient and less likely to lead to a binge. For the anorexic individual food has become associated with anxiety. The patient requires practice for her anxiety responses to subside and for the physical and social reinforcemnt involved in preparing and eating a meal to take their place. Research into the eating behavior of normal subjects has consistently shown that there is a facilitatory effect on eating by groups, particularly mixed gender groups.[39] Eating with others may provide more encouragement, support, and modelling than eating alone. The patient should be encouraged to eat out frequently; initially this should be with the therapist, but later also with family and friends.

Clothes Shopping

Since many treatment facilities keep patients in their night clothes during the first part of treatment, the clothes which they brought to the hospital with them may not fit when they finally come to put them on again. The trying on of clothes for the first time after considerable weight gain may be traumatic for the patient. Clothes may need to be altered or new clothes purchased. The occupational therapist should accompany the patient out from the hospital on her first trip to buy clothes. The opportunity can be used to examine how the patient tries to select the correct size, and she can be helped to work through the state of almost panic upon realizing that she is now a size 12 when she wished to be a size 8. As this may be the first time out of the hospital for some time, the patient will have to deal with presenting a new "fat" self in public. The patient will often feel that people are watching her and the therapist can be on hand to help the patient examine the validity of these thoughts.

Teaching Behavioral Strategies

Even when the teaching of behavioral strategies is undertaken by a psychologist, the occupational therapist should be aware of and reinforce this treatment approach in the anorexic patient's daily life. Examples of possible strategies for use with bulimic anorexics are: "Don't eat or drink other than in the company of others", "only eat set meals", and "decide what is to be eaten before beginning to eat". The most useful forms of coping strategies which can be taught appear to be those which either directly or indirectly reduce the availability of food. In addition, engaging in behavior incompatible with bingeing may also be useful, particularly at difficult times of the day such as in the evening.
Other possibly useful strategies are:

1. encouraging the patient to keep a food diary,
2. encouraging the patient to write a daily record of dysfunctional thoughts,
3. teaching the patient stress management techniques.

The Occupational Therapist may also make a home visit in order to help patients work out a particular problem, e.g., storing food or cooking meals. The learning of coping strategies in the patient's own home has obvious advantages for generalization.

Social Skills

Most individuals who suffer from anorexia nervosa appear socially adept. However, a closer look reveals that these patients are often not fulfilling their needs in social relationships. The improvement of social skills is an aim of many occupational therapy groups. Nevertheless it is useful to have a group specifically designed to get at more problematic areas of social functioning such as going to a party or being asked out by members of the opposite sex.[5] The goals of the social skills group include expression of clear, congruent, messages and examination of thinking. Techniques of assertion, self awareness, values clarification and role playing are used. Video equipment is often useful in this setting. Although good in other areas some patients social skills fail around food. It is as though the anxiety associated with eating prevents the patient from doing anything other than withdrawing. The patient fails to participate in any active way and does not enjoy herself. To overcome this problem the occupational therapist can introduce food to the social skills group. Sending out for pizza is a good example.

Relaxation

The possible advantages of relaxation training are numerous. Various relaxation techniques can be used such as deep breathing, visualization and contract-relax methods.[40,41] The most important benefits which might be derived from relaxation training by anorexic patients are briefly summarized below:

1. Reduction in anxiety levels,
2. Increased competency in dealing with stress,
3. Avoiding unwanted behaviors which appear to depend (at least in part) on stress, e.g., bingeing,
4. Increased self esteem as a result of increased control over stress reactions,
5. Improved interpersonal relationships.

Many anorexic patients are hyperactive and show an inability to relax. Generally anorexic patients seem to have difficulty in understanding and responding to the messages which they receive from their body.[7] Biofeedback can be used to help the patient become more aware of her body and develop awareness of internal stimuli. Biofeedback helps the patient gain healthy control by providing precise and easily understandable information about bodily functioning.[42] Some patients may object to becoming relaxed because of a fear of losing control. The occupational therapist must be prepared to discuss this and deal with issues which arise for the patient when relaxed. As patients are often at their most anxious before and after meals it may be appropriate to schedule the relaxation sessions at these times. Patients should be encouraged to note when they become tense throughout the day and to use the techniques which they have learned in sessions at these times.

Exercise

Exercise sessions are helpful in teaching patients how to moderate their level of activity as well as providing an opportunity for toning, strengthening and cardiac reconditioning. The therapist can assist the patient in noting bodily changes and sensations which signal sufficient exercise.[20] The therapist also helps the patient examine her normal daily routines in relation to an exercise program. The more exercise the patient's general activities involve, the less she will need to engage in additional exercises of any sort. The patient can also practise adjusting her food intake to maintain a constant weight. As the anorexic is typically hospitalized in a depleted and tense state her general endurance and overall strength may be low. Cardiac performance should be monitored at all times. This is especially important for patients with metabolic abnormalities, particularly those with hypokalaemia associated with chronic vomiting, as they are known to be prone to severe arhythmias including ventricular fibrilation.

Body Image Distortion

The effects of possible treatment approaches for body image distortion in anorexia nervosa are still unknown. Two avenues are available to the therapist. The first is to continue to present to the patient information on her actual body size by, for example, the use of video equipment, in order to help generate a more realistic appraisal of body size. The second strategy is to concentrate on examining the subjective meaning of body size for the patient. Gottheil et al.[43] reported successful treatment of an anorexic patient's denial of thinness by repeatedly confronting her with motion pictures of her emaciated body. Many therapists however prefer to approach the problem indirectly.[44] Garner et al.[38] among others, suggest that rather than attempting to alter misperceptions directly, the therapist should help the patient change how she interprets them. The patient may for example be taught that they are manifestations of illness and that they should be ignored in favor of other more objective criteria such as the opinion of a trusted friend.[25]

EXPRESSIVE TECHNIQUES

The following discussion of creative and expressive techniques is selective. The exclusion of such approaches as music, dance, and drama therapy is not intended as a comment on their value, although the appropriateness of different techniques will vary between treatment settings.

Creative Media

Crafts such as pottery, weaving, leather work and printing, particularly when conducted in a group, require skills and involve self expression.[5] The skill of the occupational therapist comes in adapting the activity to the needs of the patient. So for example some activities are more isolating than others, some require a lot of concentration, some not so much. Working in pairs or on projects requires varying levels of accommodation to the needs or wishes of others,[45] some activities require high levels of frustration tolerance, some provide easy success and the joy of creation. Activity diverts attention away from the self protection which is involved in the denial of feeling. Patients who deny a particular emotion, e.g., frustration, will often make their feelings perfectly clear to themselves by the way they handle the clay or the leather work. Like any activity, craft activity can be used cognitively to examine thoughts and styles of thinking. The patient's reactions to failure and frustration can be examined and adaptive coping techniques developed.

Art Therapy

When using art as an expressive medium the quality of the art work is much less important than the act of production, and the way the art helps the patient see herself and her ideas in concrete form. Art can be used in a number of different ways. Martin gives the example of a therapist employing hand and finger painting, and color collages early in treatment in order to help the patient express moods and emotions. Later more threatening material may be dealt with by the therapist's suggesting titles such as ''How I feel at target weight'', ''How I see my family'', ''What I would like to be'', in order to tap more complex ideas and feelings.[5]

Creative Movement

The goals of the creative movement group are to help the anorexic patient increase self awareness through movement, and identify and express feelings. Many psychotherapeutic approaches have stressed the integration of mind and body. Patients may be thought of as repressing feelings by muscular tensions. These psychological repressions restrict personal growth and development, just as the patient's abstinence from food prevents physical growth and development. In many ways a person's sense of self is perceived through their body. The creative movement group focusses on the individual's experience of their body. Patients are encouraged to use their bodies as a means of self expression. Many patients report hating their bodies and being disgusted by them. The group focusses on trying to help the patient feel good about their body by exploring these emotions. Creative movement helps the patient develop a simultaneous awareness of self and environment. It has also been proposed that movement helps the individual to integrate various aspects of the self including various levels of awareness, memory, sensations, and emotions.

CONCLUSION

This paper has presented a model for the treatment of anorexia nervosa. Special attention has been paid to the importance of continuing assessment involving the participation of both the therapist and the patient. Involving the patient in her treatment is probably the most essential requirement, and the one which is hardest to obtain. We have discussed the cognitive behavioral approach as a model for the therapist, and how it can help her link her treatment of the patient's thoughts, emotions and behavior. Although the occupational therapist's level of involvement with this population has been increasing there is still underutilization of the occupational therapists skills and this is reflected in the literature. Occupational therapists are still having to educate those involved in health care at all levels, from the unit administrators and treatment teams to the patient herself.

REFERENCES

1. Palmer, R.L., "Anorexia Nervosa". In Granville-Grossman, K., (ed). "Recent Advances in Clinical Psychiatry", No. 4. Edinburgh, Churchill Livingstone, 1982.

2. Theander, S., Anorexia Nervosa; A Psychiatric Investigation of 94 Female Patients. Acta Psychiatrica Scandinavica, Supplement 214. 1970.

3. Kendall, R.E., Hall, D.J., Hailey, A. and Babigian, H.M. "The Epidemiology of Anorexia Nervosa". Psychological Medicine, Vol 3. No 2. 1973.

4. Deusen, J.V., Allen, M.E., "Is there Perceptual-Motor Dysfunction in Anorexia nervosa? Suggestions for Research by therapists". In Press.

5. Martin, J.E., "Anorexia Nervosa: a Disorder of Weight". The British Journal of Occupational Therapy, Vol 41, No 9, 1978.

6. Giles, G.M. and Chng, C.L., "Occupational therapy in the Treatment of Anorexia Nervosa: A Contractual-Coping Approach". The British Journal of Occupational Therapy, Vol 47, No 5, 1984.

7. Bruch, H., "Eating disorders, Obesity, Anorexia Nervosa and the Person Within". New York, Basic Books, 1973.

8. Leon, G.R. "Anorexia Nervosa: The Question of Treatment Emphasis". Behavioral Medicine.

9. Lang, P.J. "Behavior Therapy with a Case of Anorexia Nervosa". In Ullman, L.P. and Krasmer, L. (ed). Case Studies in Behavior Modification. New York. Holt, Rinehard and Winston. 1965.

10. Argyle, M., Trower, P.E. and Bryant, B.M. "Explorations in the Treatment of Neuroses and Personality Disorders by Social Skills Training". British Journal of Medical Psychology. 47. 1974.

11. Pillay, M. and Crisp, A.H. "The Impact of Social Skills Training within an Established In-Patient Treatment Programme for Anorexia Nervosa". British Journal of Psychiatry. 139. 1981.

12. Fries, H. "Studies on Secondary Amenorrhea, Anorectic Behavior and Body Image Perception: Importance for the Early Recognition of Anorexia Nervosa". In Vigersky, R.A., (ed). "Anorexia Nervosa". New York, Raven Press, 1977.

13. Slade, P.D., and Russell, G.F.M. "Awareness of Body Dimensions in Anorexia Nervosa: Cross-Sectional and Longitudinal Studies". Psychological Medicine. 3. 1973.

14. Button, E.J., Fransella, F. and Slade, P.D. "A Reappraisal of Body Perception Disturbance in Anorexia Nervosa". Psychological Medicine. 7. 1977.

15. Wingate, B.A. and Christie, M.J. "Ego-Strength and Body Image in Anorexia Nervosa". Journal of Psychosomatic Research. 22. 1978.

16. Garfinkel, P.E., Moldofsky, H. and Garner, D.M. "The Outcome of Anorexia Nervosa: Significance of Clinical Features, Body Image, and Behaviour Modification". In Vigersky, R.A., "Anorexia Nervosa". New York, Raven Press, 1977.

17. Morgan, H.G. and Russell, G.F.M. "Value of Family Background and Clinical Features as Predictors of Long term Outcome in Anorexia Nervosa: 4 Year Follow Up Study of 41 Patients". Psychological Medicine. 5. 1975.

18. Hsu, L.K.G., Crisp, A.H. and Harding, B. "Outcome of Anorexia Nervosa". Lancet 1. 1979.

19. Morgan, H.G., Purgold, J. and Welbourne, J. "Management and Outcome in Anorexia Nervosa: A Standardized Prognostic Study". British Journal of Psychiatry, 143. 1983.

20. Holgren, S., Sohlberg, S., Berg, E., Johansson, B.M., Norring, C., and Rosmark, B. "Phase 1 Treatment of the Chronic and Previously Treated Anorexic Bulimia Patient". International Journal of Eating Disorders, Vol 3. No 2, 1984.

21. Russell, G.F.M., "General Management of Anorexia Nervosa and Difficulties in Assessing the Efficacy of Treatment". In Vigersky, R.A. (ed). "Anorexia Nervosa". New York, Raven Press, 1977.

22. Sours, J., "The Anorexia Nervosa Syndrome: Phenomenologic and Psychodynamic Components". Psychiatric Quarterly 43, 1969.

23. Minuchin, S., Rosman, B.L. and Baker, L. "Psychosomatic Families: Anorexia Nervosa in Context". Cambridge, Harvard University Press, 1978.

24. Agras, S. and Werne, J. "Behavior Modification in Anorexia nervosa: Research Foundations". In Vigersky, R.A., (ed). "Anorexia Nervosa". New York, Raven Press, 1977.

25. Garner, D.M. and Bemis, K.M., "A Cognitive-Behavioural Approach to Anorexia Nervosa". Cognitive Therapy and Research, Vol 6, No. 2, 1982.

26. Giles, G.M., "Anorexia Nervosa and Bulimia: An Activity-Oriented Approach". American Journal of Occupational Therapy. In press.

27. Branch, C.H.H. and Eurman, L.J., "Social Attitudes Towards Patients With Anorexia Nervosa". American Journal of Psychiatry. 173. 1980.

28. Booth, D.A., "Satiety and Appetitie Are Conditioned Reactions". Psychosomatic Medicine 39, 76, 1977.

29. Bruch, H., "Hunger and Instinct". Journal of Nervous and Mental Diseases. 149, 91. 1969.

30. Herman, C.P. and Mack, D., "Restrained and Unrestrained Eating". Journal of Personality. 43. 1975.

31. Cauwels, J.M., "Bulimia: The Binge-Purge Compulsion". New York. Doubleday, 1983.

32. Pickar, D., Cohen, M.R., Naber, D., and Cohen, R.M. "Clinical Studies of the Endogenous Opioid System". Biological Psychiatry, Vol 17, No. 11. 1982.

33. Beluzzi, J.D., and Stein, L. "Enkephalin may Mediate Euphoria and Drive Reward". Nature, Vol 266, No. 5602. 1977.

34. Slade, P., "Towards a Functional Analysis of Anorexia Nervosa and Bulimia Nervosa". British Journal Of Clinical Psychology, No 21, 1982.

35. Kanfer, F.H., and Saslow, G. "Behavioral Diagnosis in Behavior Therapy: Appraisal and Status". Franks, C.M., (ed). New York. McGraw-Hill. 1969.

36. Beck, A.T., "Cognitive Therapy and the Emotional Disorders". New York, International Universities Press, 1976.

37. Fairburn, M.A., "The place of the Cognitive Behavioral Approach in the Management of Bulimia". In Darby, P.L., Garfinkel, P.E., Garner, D.M., and Coscina, D.V. (eds). Anorexia Nervosa. New York, Alan Liss. 1983.

38. Garner, D.M., Garfinkle, P.E., and Bemis, K.M. "A Multidimensional Psychotherapy for Anorexia Nervosa". International Journal of Eating Disorders, Vol 1. No 2, 1982.

39. Klesges, R.C., Bartsch, D., Norwood, J.D., Kautzman, D. and Haugrud, S. "The Effects of Selected Social and Enviromental Variables on the Eating Behavior of Adults in the Natural Enviroment". International Journal of Eating Disorders, Vol 3. No 2, 1984.

40. Jacobson, E. "Progressive Relaxation". University of Chicago Press. Chicago. 1938.

41. Shultz, J.M. and Luthe, W. "Autogenic Therapy". Vol 1. Autogenic Methods. New York. Grune and Stratton. 1969.

42. Mckee, M.G. and Kiffer, J.F. "Clinical Biofeedback Therapy in the Treatment of Anorexia. In Gross, M. (ed). Anorexia Nervosa. Collamore Press. 1982.

43. Gottheil, E., Backup, C.E. and Cornelison, F.S. "Denial and Self Image Confrontation in a case of Anorexia Nervosa". The Journal of Nervous and Mental Diseases. 148. 1969.

44. Lucas, A.R., Duncan, J.W. and Piens, V. "The Treatment of Anorexia Nervosa" American Journal of Psychiatry. Vol. 133 No 9. 1976.

45. Mosey, A.C. "Activities Therapy". London, Raven Press, 1973.

Treatment of the Hospitalized Eating Disorder Patient

David Roth, PhD

ABSTRACT. Research and understanding of the development and expression of anorexia and bulimia have increased dramatically over the past decade. Causal agents and treatment of eating disorders are reviewed. An inpatient therapy program describes the unique needs of eating disorder patients and two key facets, the inpatient milieu and the consolidated group therapy program.

Contemporary interest in eating disorders is rooted in the exceptionally perceptive and thought provoking studies of Hilde Bruch (1978, 1982). While Bruch's investigations can be traced back to the 1940's, it has only been within the past decade that the eating disorder literature has burgeoned. With the rapid growth of investigations in this area, researchers are increasingly able to identify the multiplicity of factors which place one at risk for developing and sustaining an eating disorder. Expanded understanding of eating disorders is paralleled by the birth and maturation of current day treatment regimes and specialty eating disorder units. Clinicians, cognizant of the complexity of these disorders, are making use of the biopsychosocial intervention which includes treatment of the patient's psyche, body, and family.

This paper reviews various factors believed to be causally related to the development, onset, and maintenance of eating disorders. An inpatient eating disorder program with emphasis on milieu and group interventions is described.

CAUSAL MODEL OF EATING DISORDERS

A multidimensional analysis is needed to understand why a particular group of individuals evidence a sustained pattern of symp-

Dr. Roth is Director of the Inpatient Eating Disorder Program and Director of the Outpatient Eating Disorder Clinic at The Sheppard and Enoch Pratt Hospital in Towson, Maryland 21204.

67

toms. Crisp (1984) noted that eating disorders represent a "coming together of many determining factors, which can be expressed in cultural, social, experiential, and somatic dimensions" (p. 209). A useful heuristic (Weiner, 1977) begins with an examination of the factors which make one vulnerable for the development of a given disorder. These can be referred to as *predispositional* factors. The comprehensive theory sets out to identify conditions or *precipitants* which provoke the manifestation of a given symptom cluster in the vulnerable individual. The theoretician must also articulate a set of variables which *perpetuate* a pattern of symptoms over a period of time.

Eating disorders represent a heterogeneous grouping of syndromes (Strober, 1983). As the field is still in its infancy, the following discussion of predisposing, precipitating, and perpetuating factors will at times refer to anorexia nervosa, at other times to bulimia, and occasionally to the generic family of eating disorders. An extensive review is available in Garner and Garfinkel (1982).

Predispositional Factors

Interpersonal transactions, affective experiences, and activities of daily living are strongly influenced by the beliefs we hold about ourselves and our world. High risk takers are often individuals who view themselves as having extraordinary abilities and/or view their jobs as being challenging but not exceptionally dangerous. Armed with these beliefs, the mountain climber will traverse a steep peak, "knowing" that it is only a moderately threatening task which (s)he is more than equipped to handle. Analogously, phobia clinics regularly treat patients who perceive themselves as being quite fragile (e.g., agoraphobics) and/or see their worlds as being very dangerous (e.g., plane or bridge phobics). Belief systems are laid down early in life and are shaped, molded, and modified throughout the course of one's life. The genesis of an eating disorder becomes clearer as one examines the premorbid pattern of beliefs, expectations, and attitudes which are held by the pre-anorectic or pre-bulimic person.

The development of anorexia is closely linked to the sense of ineffectiveness and worthlessness which these girls hold about themselves (Bruch, 1978; Garfinkel and Garner, 1982; Selvini-Palazzoli, 1974). The anorectic individual experiences herself as being out of control and a captive of forces within her family and broader social spheres. Life's problems, whether they be at school, with peers, or on a part-time job are interpreted in a manner which is consistent with the individual's core belief structure. These difficulties are seen as being derivatives of personal inadequacies that are most likely incorrectable without external intervention. Anorectic persons devalue themselves by setting unrealistically high expectations which Mahoney (1974) has referred to as a "cycle of inflationary self-evaluations." By requiring oneself to perform perfectly, the anorectic discounts performances which would otherwise have been viewed as accomplishments. This process is doubly damning when one considers that maintaining unachievable perfectionistic standards ultimately reinforces the pre-anorectic's belief that she is a grand-scale failure.

Many of the symptoms seen in anorectic patients can be understood in light of their core belief system. First, restrictive eating, highly structured food rituals, and excessive exercising can be conceptualized as a way of providing these individuals with both a sense of worth and control. Rather than being a "nobody," they are transformed into "olympic" quality dieters. Bruch (1982) wrote, " . . . these girls feel helpless and ineffective in conducting their own lives, and the severe discipline over their bodies represents a desperate effort to ward off panic about being powerless" (p. 1532). Second, the anorectic's efforts to diet are further exacerbated in that subgroup of girls who evidence a vulnerability to overestimating their body size (Garner, Garfinkel, Stanker, and Moldofsky, 1976). Third, anorectic individuals' tendency to turn to others for external validation and their distrust of internal affective states can be traced back to an overriding belief that they are inadequate and ineffective. Finally, the schizoid-like posture which is frequently demonstrated by the anorectic patient is also directly related to their underlying beliefs. One often hears these individuals say that they will not only be unable to meet other people's expectations, but that they will eventually be "found out" as unworthy people and subsequently rejected.

Although the anorectic person has received attention from both the popular and scientific presses, there is a noticeable dearth of literature concerning the family dynamics which place them at risk for developing an eating disorder. Research in this area is still in its infancy because of such factors as familial resistance to being studied, small sample size, use of poorly validated instrumentation, and inherent difficulty in differentiating between familial patterns which predate the onset of an eating disorder and those which are a reaction to the illness. However, progress is being made in identification of discrete, dysfunctional intrafamilial patterns. Researchers are beginning to isolate differential subtypes of familial pathology (Andersen, 1985; Garfinkel and Garner, 1982; Johnson and Flack, 1984; Strober, Salkin, Burroughs, and Morrell, 1982).

Concerns about weight and appearance are often passed directly from parent to child and from one child to another. Families of eating disorder patients frequently display an overemphasis upon thinness, firmness, attractiveness, and socially appropriate eating habits (Kalucy, Crisp, Harding, 1977; Yager, 1984). These attributes are apt to be equated by the family with self-worth, self-control, and self-discipline. Hence, the pre-anorectic child is raised to believe that in order to be "all right" as a person she must "eat right and look right."

The seeds of an eating disorder go well beyond over-attention to one's body. Minuchin and his colleagues (Minuchin, Rosman, and Baker, 1978) have articulated four transactional patterns which are frequently seen in anorectic families. First, anorectic families tend to be over-involved or, in other words, *enmeshed* in one another's lives. Boundaries around subsystems (e.g., the parents) are often violated, there is an absence of privacy, and it is expected that intimate feelings, thoughts, and experiences will be openly shared. Second, parents of anorectic girls are apt to be *overprotective* of their children. The threshold for "rescuing" their kids from perceived threats tends to be relatively low. Third, one is likely to find these families circumventing direct confrontations, and interparental problems may be denied, derailed, and displaced onto the anorectic child. Harmony, or its facsimile, is sought after by these families who can be described as conflict avoiders. Finally, the three aforementioned communicational and transactional patterns are often inaccessible to change. The rules guiding family relationships tend to be rigidly adhered to across situations and developmental epochs. Thus, the late adolescent is protected as vigorously as the prepubertal child. The observations of the Minuchin group have received support from other researchers (Bruch, 1978, Crisp, 1984; Dally, 1969; Garfinkel and Garner, 1982; Selvini-Palazzoli, 1974).

Early and prolonged home-based learning experiences fail to prepare the pre-anorectic child for the pressure and stresses which they will encounter later in life. Their development of a sense of autonomy and self-sufficiency has been blocked by their parents' intrusiveness and overprotectiveness. Bruch (1982) describes this process in a patient who believed that "my mother always knew how I felt. I never thought that it mattered what I said I felt" (p. 1534). These children are further thwarted in their efforts to gain effective control within their social sphere by being exposed to parental role models who themselves are deficient in problems solving skills. Anorectic children learn that they need to turn to their bodies to gain both self-worth and self-esteem.

The contribution of social mores to the development of both anorexia and bulimia has been amply documented. Women in our culture are inundated with the message that their bodies are key determinants of their "position in the world" (Orbach, 1984). The media impresses upon women that small busts, slight hips, and the Victorian eighteen inch waist represent the ideal body form. One can begin her day with a televised aerobics lesson, go on to attend a weight watcher's or diet workshop class, and end her day with a health salad and a viewing of Jane Fonda's videotaped workout. A plethora of studies attest to the concern which young women have about their bodies (Crisp, 1984; Nylander, 1971; Crisp, Palmer and Kalucy, 1972). Moreover, the impact upon women of shifting cultural values is supported by research demonstrating that a rise in the incidence of eating disorders is paralleled by changes in the shape of Miss America Pageant contestants and Playboy centerfolds (Garner, Garfinkel, Schwartz, and Thompson, 1980).

Cultural expectations predispose young girls to develop eating disorders in a second, albeit more subtle, manner. Eating disorders are more prevalent in girls who come from middle and upper social class backgrounds (Garfinkel and Garner, 1982) which place a high value upon exceptional achievement and perfectionistic-like performance. Rigorous adherence to these standards is apt to result in a series of perceived failures and to reinforce the beliefs that one is worthless and ineffective. A young girl is now faced with an abundance of options to choose from. Shall she enter the professions and, if so, then which one? Should she postpone sexual intimacies until she is in "love" or should she experiment whenever an opportunity is available? The adult world is a frightening place when one believes that there are too many choices, lack of preparation for making them, and only an "A" quality performance is acceptable. Retreating into childhood is one solution to this dilemma.

Evidence suggests that bulimic individuals manifest substantially different patterns of behavior, cognition, and affect than anorectic individuals manifest. Bulimics have been characterized as being impulsive, experiencing quite dramatic shifts in their mood, feeling as if they are out of control, and viewing the world through a dichotomous, all-or-none perspective (Beaumont, George, Smart, 1976; Garfinkel and Garner, 1984; Norman and Herzog, 1983; Pyle, Mitchell, and Eckert, 1981; Strober, 1981). These individuals are also apt to be at a significant risk for affective disorders (Hudson, Laffer, and Pope, 1982; Strober, Salkin, Burroughs, and Morrell, 1982). Paralleling their internal chaos, bulimics often come from families which are disorganized, imbued with conflict and parental discord, and are relatively unstructured, and noncohesive (Beaumont et al., 1976; Garfinkel and Garner, 1984; Johnson and Flach, 1984; Strober et al., 1982).

The chaos and turbulence of the bulimic's affective intrapsychic, and interpersonal spheres can be viewed as placing them at risk for the development of an eating disorder. Bulimics describe cycles of bingeing, purging, and restricting as overt manifestations of their internal fragmentation. By gorging themselves, bulimics can focus their attention away from paralyzing thoughts and, at times, can "safely" act out their impulses. The sedative effects of a binge serve the same function of affect regulation as would alcohol or drugs.

The frequent finding that bulimics tend to be premorbidly obese points to another potential risk factor (Wardle and Beinart, 1981). The bulimic individual may be predisposed for being overweight, that is, her/his "set point," or biological weight, may be substantially higher than the cultural "set point." The cravings to eat which frequently precede a binge may at times be secondary to the discrepancy between the bulimic's ideal and biological weights. Supporting this position are the anecdotal reports by patients who frequently find themselves bingeing after a period of restrictive fasting.

Precipitants

Explanations of the onset of a given symptom pattern are often derived from a simple cause and effect model. The juxtaposition, in time and space, of a stressor (e.g., death of a wife stressor) and a symptom (e.g., grief of a husband) are frequently interpreted as if the stressor itself caused or precipitated the symptom. Processes internal to the individual which mediate between the stressor and the symptom are absent from this analysis. The subjective meaning of the stressor and the act of deciding how to cope with the perceived state of affairs are lacking. Comprehensive analysis of the onset of an eating disorder must extend beyond life events and symptomatic expression to include an examination of the cognitive linkage between these events.

Anorexia nervosa represents a functional, yet maladaptive, reaction to the stressors inherent in adolescence. Onset of this disorder typically occurs in the beginning, middle, and late stages of puberty (Halmi, Casper, Eckert, Goldberg, and Davis, 1979). It is during this time that the growing child is faced with a number of stressing developmental tasks (Crisp, 1980). On one level the child must move from the relatively safe and protected world of her parents into a more complex, demanding and unpredictable external world. At home, they are allowed to be dependent; yet outside of this "cocoon," they are required to become independent. Correspondingly, adolescence is a time when one moves away from a strict adherence to their parents' values in order to incorporate the mores of their peers. At home they were "unconditionally" valued, but in their new social sphere they can and will be rejected. They are faced with new choices regarding their sexuality in which they must decide when and whether to date, to pet, and to make love. Ultimately, high school comes to an end and these young women are confronted with choices about leaving home—both psychologically and physically. As Yager (1984) has commented, "All these events are within the ordinary vicissitudes of adolescent life" (p. 436).

The anorectic's decision to restrictively fast can be seen as a means of avoiding the developmental tasks of adolescence which they believe they are unequipped to tackle. In other words, anorexia may represent a "biological solution to an existential problem . . . " (Crisp, 1984). Anorexia provides these girls with something they can excel at. At the same time it enables them to avoid stressors which would further weaken their already limited sense of self-esteem.

Precipitants of bulimia are less certain than those of anorexia. Investigators have primarily focused upon the role played by dieting and affective-interpersonal distress. Studies conducted by a number of independent research groups indicate that the binge-purge cycle quite regularly follows a period of intense restrictive dieting (Boskind-Lodahl, 1976; Wooley and Wooley, 1982; Pyle et al., 1981). Clinical observations reveal that many of these individuals view their diets in an all-or-none manner. The smallest breach of their diet is perceived to be a major violation which merits an all-out binge. Coupled with this pattern of thinking is the belief that by vomiting or taking laxatives, they can "safely" fulfill their cravings without fear of weight gain.

Other researchers have found that bulimia is precipitated by significant interpersonal stress (Loro and Orleans, 1981; Pyle et al., 1981; Strober, 1984) and/or intense affective distress (Johnson and Larson, 1982). In these circumstances a binge may serve both an integrative and regulative function. Food provides a focal point. Experientially, it helps the bulimic seemingly gain control over internal and external chaos. They can feel full rather than empty, lonely, and depressed. Additionally, they can distract themselves from thinking self-deprecatory and catastrophic thoughts. Given the disorganization and conflict they have experienced in their families, food, rather than people, is seen as providing the safest refuge.

Perpetuating Factors

Bulimia and anorexia represent a rather formidable challenge to the mental health system. It is relatively common to find eating disorder patients with a chronic history of seriously impaired functioning. Quite recently, Jane Fonda openly acknowledged having been bulimic for well over twenty years. Moreover, many have kept their symptom patterns so well concealed that even their spouses and therapists are surprised to learn about the psychopathology. To understand the enduring nature of eating disorders one needs to examine the interaction among multiple biological, social, and psychological factors.

Eating disorders follow a self-perpetuating course, and the biological mechanisms involved in this chain of events are keenly illustrated in both anorexia and bulimia. The anorectic who has reached a starvation weight presents symptomatology which is secondary to the starvation and reinforcing of the primary pathology. For instance, it is known that starving individuals become preoccupied with food, obsessional, experience mood lability, impaired concentration, and indecisiveness (Keys, Brezek, Henschel, Mickelsen, Taylor, 1950). These same symptoms have a "reverberating" effect on the anorectic by exacerbating their fears of losing control with food and potentiating their sense of ineffectiveness. Delayed gastric emptying time results in an exaggerated sense of fullness and consequently engenders further restricting (Garfinkel,

1974; Saleh and Lebwahl, 1980). The alternating and chaotic cycle of bingeing, purging, and restricting which is symptomatic of bulimia is apt to have analogous consequences. These individuals are inclined to experience episodes of intense hunger and thereby "prime" themselves for a subsequent binge.

The influence which interpersonal forces have upon the course of an eating disorder is well documented in the clinical literature. One need only turn to their local college to observe the pernicious effect of *social validation*. The bulimics who attend the SEPH outpatient clinic readily articulate that many of their friends, even roommates, are practicing bulimics. By reference to the habits of their peers, they can sanction the continuation of their own eating disorder. Similarly, anorectics are often praised for their weight loss (Branch and Eurman, 1980). Compliments regarding their appearance, discipline and "will power" are liberally received at the beginning of their diet and continue, at a greatly reduced frequency, until they have reached a cachexic appearance. Rarely are anorectic persons refused admission to the swim team, gym class, and other formal exercise groups. Their teachers "quietly" collude with their maintenance of the anorectic stance. It is important to note that families of anorectics often perpetuate the illusion of well-being by acceding to patients' requests for premature discharge from inpatient treatment programs (Vandereycken and Pierloot, 1983). The importance of having a sick child in the family is frequently underscored by the deterioration of a parent as the anorectic's illness remits (Crisp, Harding, and McGuiness, 1974).

Belief systems and philosophies of living are quite resistant to modification. Unaltered patterns of thinking perpetuate the same patterns of behavior. The core assumptions which eating disordered patients hold about themselves, their relationships, and their position in the world tend to be firmly rooted cognitive schematas. The all-or-none thinking and the beliefs of worthlessness and inadequacy which initially predisposed these people to develop an eating disorder foster the repetitive manifestation of eating disordered symptoms.

For many patients, the underlying predispositional beliefs become part of a broader self-perpetuating cognitive system; hence, the eating disorder which was once ego-dystonic becomes their core identity. It provides them with a sense of purpose and specialness which they will fight to preserve. They knowingly describe themselves as "bulimics" and "anorectics," although earlier in their illness, they were people "suffering from" bulimia or anorexia. At this stage, cognitive operations and behavioral planning stem from the central assumption that they are eating disordered. Fasting and hunger are interpreted as ego enhancing signs of self-control, discipline and accomplishments. These individuals will attend eating disorder groups in order to share strategies for restricting or purging in the same way great chefs exchange their favorite recipes. Everyday problems of living are seen as if they were problems of thinness, firmness, and appearance. Anxiety about what you say to a date is viewed as anxiety over being too fat for the date. Eating disorder symptoms become their primary tool for coping with life's difficulties.

INPATIENT TREATMENT: MILIEU AND GROUPS

Effective treatment of the hospitalized eating disorder patient necessitates a truly collaborative, multidisciplinary approach. Depending upon their unique needs, eating disorder patients recieve a variety of psychological, biological, and interpersonal therapies. Because of space limitations, only two facets of the overall treatment regime—the inpatient milieu and the therapy groups—are described.

The integrated inpatient-outpatient treatment program at the Sheppard Pratt Hospital differentiates between long and short-range therapeutic goals. During the average 3-4 month hospitalization, patients concentrate on attaining the following objectives.

Eating disorder patients require nutritional rehabilitation, normalization of their eating patterns, and frequently, weight restoration. They need to clearly grasp the role which this illness assumes in their life. We attempt to help them understand how dysfunctional thinking, disturbed interpersonal relationships, and impaired health perpetuate their anorexia and/or bulimia. They are encouraged to supplant faulty habits with a more adaptive, self-enhancing system of beliefs and style of relating. The hospital is an exceedingly structured, supportive, and artificial environment. A bridge between the therapeutic "work" accomplished in the hospital and that to be continued "in vivo" involves helping transplant important skills to the external world.

Inpatient treatment begins with the preadmission interview when the patient and her family meet with the program director, the social worker, and a member of the nursing staff. During this interview, staff, patient, and family collectively determine the suitability of admission to the treatment program. Only voluntary patients are accepted to the program. The patient's commitment to recovery and their clinical-medical status are accorded equal weight in making this decision. The comprehensive nature of the eating disorder treatment regime and its rigors is described to the prospective patient. The possibility of refeeding edema, the likelihood that families will receive frantic phone calls concerning premature discharge, and the importance of family involvement in treatment are openly discussed. No pretense is made that inpatient treatment will effect a complete "cure" of one's eating disorder. Patients are cautioned that hospitalization is but one component of a broad-scale, multisequential treatment plan and that they will need to continue in outpatient treatment.

Milieu

Fundamental to attaining the aforementioned short-range goals is the use of a structured and supportive inpatient milieu. Eating disorder patients move through a three phase operantly based treatment program. Weight gain for the anorectic and inhibition of bingeing/purging behavior for the bulimic are contingently consequated with inceasing periods of free time. Blocks of free time not only reinforce the enactment of nutritionally adaptive eating patterns but also provide the patient with an opportunity to develop, practice, and overlearn healthy strategies for coping with intrapsychic and interpersonal distress.

Patients are admitted into phase one of the eating disorder program. While in this phase, they are routinely observed throughout the day by members of the nursing staff. Observations are made while the patient is using the toilet, showering and eating. It is explained to patients that they are *not* being policed. Rather, in recognizing that their eating behavior is currently out of control, staff endeavor to help them regain responsible control. Individuals are strongly encouraged to regularly discuss their anxiety about weight gain, fears of eating "dangerous" foods, impulses to binge or purge, and other eating related concerns with the nursing staff. Essentially, observation time is conceptualized as an opportunity for therapeutic growth.

It is during phase one that patients become quite familiar with the various "rules" and guiding philosophy of the eating disorder program. They learn that they will be weighed on Monday, Wednesday, and Friday mornings, post voiding and in hospital gown. All patients are informed of their weight and helped to examine and rethink the distorted meanings which weight has been accorded. One of the most valuable messages which is communicated from the onset of hospitalization concerns the role which patients assume in each other's treatment. Both eating disorder and non-eating disorder patients are expected to help one another develop rational beliefs and healthy life-styles. In practice, this means that patients will attempt to dissuade, not persuade, other members of their community to refrain from restrictive fasting, bingeing, and purging. Failure to report an instance of maladaptive behavior is viewed, by staff, as sanctioning this same behavior. Hence, relevant contingencies (e.g., hall restriction) are imposed upon the "rule-breaker" and their "collaborator(s)." By expecting the broader community to reinforce adaptive behavioral mores there are fewer "splits" between staff and patients, fewer efforts made by eating disorder patients to defeat (e.g., secretly bingeing) the treatment program, and greater attention to health and recovery.

Nutritional rehabilitation and normalization of eating patterns are initiated during phase one. All patients consult with the hospital's dietician about their daily meal plan. A dietary exchange program is used. Calories are de-emphasized in lieu of a balanced intake of the basic food groups (i.e., vegetables, fruits, milk, meats, fats, and breads). Each patient's daily caloric requirements are established during the first week of hospitalization and are modified in accordance with their treatment objectives. Stabilization of weight and regularization of eating patterns is a high priority goal for all patients. Only after this objective has been achieved is the issue of weight loss discussed with obese bulimics.

Refeeding for anorectics is initiated at between 1200-1500 calories per day. We begin with a diet low in lactose and lipids because of the possibility for gastric dilatation (Browning, 1977). Caloric increments are based upon the patient's age, rate of weight gain, and level of anxiety. A 2-3 pound weight gain per week is a goal. A goal weight range is established during the first week of hospitalization. The "midpoint" of this range is based upon the body weight needed to resume menstruation (Frisch and McArthur, 1974). The choice of this weight rests upon the assumption that starvation enables patients to avoid coming to terms with adult sexuality. Resumption of menstruation can be seen as a form of "in vivo" desensitization in that patients directly confront a feared developmental task. It should also be noted that the goal weight range extends ±3 pounds of the midpoint in order to both downplay obsessional attention to detail and to convey the message that weight "normally" fluctuates without a consequent loss of control.

During phases two and three, patients accrue increasingly more unobserved time and progressively higher levels of freedom, both within and outside the hospital. At this stage, treatment focuses upon the internalization of strategies for sustaining physical and mental health. Specifically, patients begin to exercise control over their daily diet. They learn how to: objectively judge the size of a serving of food, effectively use the exchange program, and plan, purchase, and prepare healthy meals. In phase three, patients eat in the cafeteria rather than on the unit under staff supervision (phases one and two). Moreover, we encourage patients to use local restaurants to gain further practice in utilizing self-control skills and anxiety-management strategies. Bulimics are given the opportunity to eat and prepare "binge" foods under their own guidance. Anorectic patients are asked to integrate, at their own discretion, at least one "feared" food into each meal. These "in vivo" experiences have the dual effects of buttressing patients' limited sense of efficacy and identifying treatment issues which merit more intensive staff supervision.

It is reasonable to expect that most eating disorder patients are apt to experience a period of symptomatic distress after they have been discharged. During phase three we help the patient develop a repertoire of relapse prevention skills. Patients are encouraged to identify periods of time, kinds of interpersonal interactions, patterns of thinking, and types of emotion which made them vulnerable for a recurrence of eating disorder symptoms. Concrete strategies are formulated for both preventing and coping with high risk situations. For example, patients are trained in the "prophylactic" art of managing and structuring their free time. Relevant cognitive and behavioral strategies are discussed in the group section. Given their penchant for all-or-none thinking, the eating disorder patient is inclined to view a brief relapse as a complete loss of control. By preparing patients for these episodes and labeling them as opportunities for further therapeutic growth, serious exacerbations of the eating disorder have been prevented.

In summary, patients require freedom from immediate supervision if they are ever to become their own therapeutic agents. Freedom implies choice of action. The eating disorder patient often fails to recognize that they regularly decide whether or not to act on an impulse to binge, purge, or restrict. To fully recover from an eating disorder one must consciously and freely choose not to behave in a self-destructive manner. Relative freedom from staff and parental pressures also forces patients to confront their motivation for sustaining and/or abstaining from eating disorder behaviors. The externally motivated patient is one who is apt to be a recidivist.

Treatment Groups

Eating disordered patients present a variety of skill deficiencies, behavioral excesses, and patterns of impaired cognitive functioning. Focused thematic treatment groups promote symptomatic remission and alleviation of underlying pathology. Somewhat greater attention will be accorded the "eating disorder" group since it serves as the hub from which most therapeutic activity evolves.

Eating Disorders Group

The eating disorder group gives each patient the chance to answer two related questions: "What role does my eating disorder play in my life?" and "What can I do about this?" The patient who uses this group effectively will be able to articulate the external and internal conditions under which they are likely to display eating disorder behavior, and the strategies which can be employed to prevent episodes of symptomatic behavior. The group tends to be here-and-now focused. Interventions and etiological formulations are generally derived from a cognitive-behavioral framework (Beck, 1976).

Group members often enter treatment with either no explanation or a relatively unidimensional explanation for their eating disorder. The introduction of cognitive constructs enables the patient to identify the complex patterns which typically elicit symptomatic behavior. At the most fundamental level, the patient is taught to look for situational, affective, and cognitive precipitants of eating disorder behavior. For example, in a recent therapy session, patients reported that they were at risk for bingeing when they *felt* hungry, sad, lonely, anxious, bored, and angry, and/or *thought* they were failures, worthless, being pressured by parents, confused about their options, and rejected by friends. Patients are helped to organize their observations in a sequential fashion and to recognize that dysfunctional thinking mediates disturbed feeling states and symptomatic behavior. Patients learn that their perceptions or thoughts of worthlessness precipitate feelings of sadness which are temporarily alleviated by bingeing. Thoughts that one's parents are trying to control them are likely to precipitate feelings of anger which may be "extinguished" through a binge.

As patients become more familiar with their intrapsychic world, they discover basic beliefs, central assumptions, or philosophy of life. The cognitive therapist believes that a dysfunctional system of basic beliefs is ultimately responsible for eating disorder behaviors. The following are common anorectic assumptions: "I must perform perfectly," "My value as a person stems from my appearance," and "I am essentially an inadequate person." With sufficient practice our patients become quite adept at identifying the relationship between symptomatic behavior, consciously experienced dysfunctional patterns of thinking, and underlying basic beliefs. Figure 1 illustrates the rather complicated and overdetermined cognitive foundation for a relatively simple eating disorder behavior, that of, excessive standing.

Recognition of the cognitive and affective antecedents to their eating disorder behavior acts as a springboard for additional therapeutic action. A summary of two cognitively-based strategies and interventions is provided. Patients often find themselves confronted with an "urge" to binge and restrict. Patients are asked to think of this feeling as a choice point and to consider delaying action upon their "urge" for at least five minutes. During their five minute break, it is recommended that patients engage in cognitive restructuring exercises and/or alternative self-enhancing activities (e.g., walk, call a friend, take a shower, etc.). Should a patient binge, we ask them to repeat this same therapeutic pattern when confronting the "urge" to purge. If they binge and purge, we encourage them to consider a realistic, not catastrophic, perspective regarding their behavior and to resume their normalized diet at the next scheduled meal. By structuring free time to include a variety of mastery and pleasure engendering activities patients are able to reduce the number of symptomatic related "urges."

Patients are frequently able to identify symptom engendering thoughts, well in advance of experiencing an urge to action and to learn to reconceptualize their thoughts as hypotheses. They are encouraged to examine both corroborative and disconfirming evidence

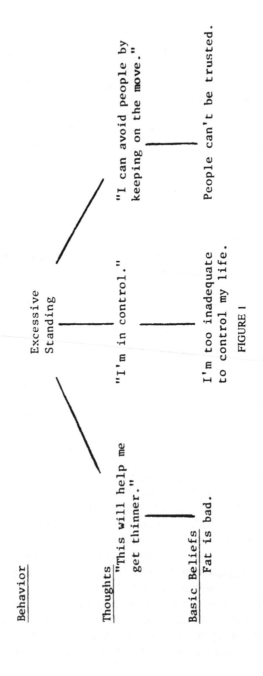

Behavior

        Excessive
        Standing

Thoughts
  "This will help me   "I'm in control."   "I can avoid people by
  get thinner."   keeping on the move."

Basic Beliefs
  Fat is bad.   I'm too inadequate   People can't be trusted.
                 to control my life.

FIGURE 1

for their thinking and generate alternative hypotheses or thoughts. Patients are also encouraged to examine the advantages and disadvantages concerning any course(s) of action which might stem from a given hypothesis or pattern of thinking. For example, a young woman who spent Saturday night in her apartment began to think, "Since I am fat no one will ever care about me. The only solution is to starve myself." Closely examining this belief, she realized that she knew a number of overweight women who were quite popular and who dated relatively often. She then decided to adopt an alternative belief, "People can like me for qualities other than my weight. I need to show more people my sensitivity and good sense of humor." Group sessions are often utilized to help patients overlearn these self-control skills.

Feelings Group

The "feelings" group utilizes cognitive principles to help foster a more differentiated understanding of affective experiences and their cognitive underpinnings. Patients with eating disorders frequently complain that they are unaware of their basic feeling states. Sadness, anxiety, and anger are frequently experienced as hunger or a sense of fatness. Through a series of structured learning experiences, patients become adept at discerning veridical affective states rather than continuing to expeience their world appetitively. Patients practice application of cognitive skills beyond the realm of their body and weight. They become cognizant of their transituational proclivity for using maladaptive cognitive patterns such as all-or-none thinking, catastrophizing, perfectionistic thinking, and discounting positive experiences. Members of this group are given a chance to examine, modify, and replace significant core beliefs concerning themselves, their social/physical world, and the future. In essence, patients are provided a safe, therapeutic context in which they can reflect upon and make decisions concerning their basic identity.

Body Movement Group

Individuals with eating orders overestimate the size of their body and/or attach negative value to various facets of their body. Patients' movement triggers self-referential feelings as shame, inadequacy, embarrassment, sexuality, aggression, and dependency.

Hence, therapeutic use of the body movement group also helps patients to correct distortions concerning their body image, to become aware of their bodily messages, and to express their feelings.

Assertion Group

The "assertion" group endeavors to provide patients with experiences which promote enhanced social comfort and a broader repertoire of adaptive interpersonal skills. Individuals with eating disorders, particularly anorectics, frequently evidence social inhibitions and find it difficult to define and to assert their rights. The paper by Mary K. Bailey, in this issue, fully describes the assertion group.

Stress Management Group

Recurrent and relatively elevated episodes of anxiety are commonly experienced by patients with eating disorders. Bingeing, restricting, and excessively exercising represent a few of their maladaptive strategies for coping with anxiety. In the "stress management" group, patients are taught a variety of anxiety reduction techniques. Skills imparted include relaxation procedures, cognitive restructuring techniques, and social support activities.

Multi-Family Group

Families of eating disorder patients receive therapeutic attention in both individual and group contexts. Relatives of patients are encouraged to attend the "multi-family group." Participation in the group provides families with pragmatic information about hospitalization and an opportunity to share and work through feelings of anger, guilt, and sadness associated with their relatives' illness. Exposure to other families with diverse intrafamilial relationships helps to highlight the disorganization, enmeshment, overprotectiveness, and impaired conflict resolution skills which are so often characteristic of the eating disorder family.

Women's Group

Social forces contribute quite directly to the formation and perpetuation of eating disorder lifestyles. The culturally defined roles which eating disorder patients ascribe to are closely examined in the women's group. Frequent topics of discussion center around such issues as body image, sexuality, femininity, and interpersonal relationships. Questions regarding autonomy and dependency are often raised by group members, and alternatives to self-denying and self-destructive cultural prescriptions are openly addressed. Since the group is composed of both eating disorder and non-eating disorder patients, there is ample opportunity to talk with women who live relatively healthy, self-enhancing lifestyles.

A number of group related procedural, conceptual, and clinical issues merit considerations. Most groups are co-led by a member of the nursing staff and a member of the professional staff. The arrangement is an exceptionally effective mechanism for coordinating and integrating various facets of the overall program, disparate observations about our patients, and a high degree of inter-member interaction. Patients are often more responsive to a given therapeutic message when it is delivered by a peer rather than by a therapist. Reinforcing group interaction allows the group to be used as the social microcosym which it represents. Sessions which are rigidly structured, allowing only for the didactic presentation of "educational" material preclude important opportunities to learn about one's social side. Interpersonal issues which routinely arise in the course of treatment concern trust, fear of rejection, competition (e.g., weight, discipline, etc.), and intimacy. Group norms can decisively influence whether patients progress or regress during their hospitalization. An avoidant, denying, and distrustful group can be rather destructive; hence, groups are oriented towards recovery and the development of active, adaptive skills for gaining control of one's life.

An important staff group is the "Eat Meet," which affords an opportunity to intensively address both patient and staff issues. First, we regularly review the progress of all patients within the eating disorder program. Clinical vignettes are shared and treatment plans are coordinated. Second, administrative decisions regarding relevant clinical policy are typically made in this group. Staff ask for clarification, reaffirmation, or modification of various facets of the overall treatment regime. Third, feelings which are aroused when working with this group of patients can be safely vented. Patients with eating disorders are prone to be rebellious, resistant to treatment, and inclined to "split" staff. By openly sharing feelings and problem solving how to respond to provocative behavior, staff mental health is preserved and divisive and nontherapeutic struggles are prevented.

In summary, research on the etiology of eating disorders will continue to examine the complex interrelationship between predisposing, precipitating, and perpetuating factors, and comprehensive understanding of the causes and nature of eating disorders will result in improved treatment interventions.

REFERENCES

Andersen, A. (1985). *Practical comprehensive treatment of anorexia nervosa and bulimia.* Baltimore: Johns Hopkins University Press.

Beaumont, P., George, G., & Smart, D. (1976). "Dieters" and "vomiters and purgers" in anorexia nervosa. *Psychological Medicine, 6,* 617-622.

Beck, A. T. (1976). *Cognitive therapy and the emotional disorders.* New York: International Universities Press.

Boskind-Lodahl, M. (1976). Cinderella's step-sisters: A feminist perspective on anorexia nervosa and bulimia. *Signs: The Journal of Women in Culture and Society, 2,* 342-356.

Branch, C. H., & Eurman, L. J. (1980). Social attitudes toward patients with anorexia nervosa. *American Journal of Psychiatry, 137,* 631-632.

Browning, C. H. (1977). Anorexia nervosa: Complications of somatic therapy. *Comprehensive Psychiatry, 18,* 399-403.

Bruch, H. (1978). *The golden cage: The enigma of anorexia nervosa.* Cambridge, Mass.: Harvard University Press.

Bruch, H. (1982). Anorexia nervosa: Therapy and theory. *American Journal of Psychiatry, 139,* 1531-1538.

Crisp, A. (1980). *Anorexia nervosa: Let me be.* London: Academic Press.

Crisp, A. (1984). The psychopathology of anorexia nervosa: Getting the "heat" out of the system. In Albert J. Stunkard & Eliot Stellar (Eds.). *Eating and its disorders.* New York: Raven Press.

Crisp, A., Harding, B., & McGuiness, G. (1974). Anorexia nervosa, psychoneurotic characteristics of parents: Relationship to prognosis, a quantitative study. *Journal of Psychosomatic Research, 18,* 167-173.

Crisp, A. H., Palmer, R. L., & Kalucy, R. S. (1976) How common is anorexia nervosa? A prevalence study. *British Journal of Psychiatry, 218,* 549-554.

Dally, P. J. (1969). *Anorexia nervosa.* New York: Greene & Stratton.

Frisch, R. E. & McArthur, J. W. (1974). Menstrual cycles: Fatness as a determinant of minimum weight necessary for their maintenance or onset. *Science, 185,* 949-951.

Garfinkel, P. (1974). Perception of hunger and satiety in anorexia nervosa. *Psychological Medicine, 4,* 309-315.

Garfinkel, P., & Garner, D. (1982). *Anorexia nervosa: A multidimensional perspective.* New York: Brunner/Mazel.

Garfinkel, P., & Garner, D. (1984). Bulimia in anorexia nervosa. In R. Hawkins, W. Fremauw, & P. Clement (Eds.). *The binge-purge syndrome.* New York: Springer.

Garner, D., Garfinkel, P., Stancer, H., & Moldofsky, H. (1976). Body image disturbances in anorexia nervosa and obesity. *Psychosomatic Medicine, 38,* 227-236.

Garner, D., Garfinkel, P., Schwartz, D., & Thompson, M. (1980). Cultural expectations of thinness in women. *Psychological Reports, 47,* 483-491.

Halmi, K., Casper, R., Eckert, E., Goldberg, S., & Davis, J. (1979). Unique features associated with age of onset of anorexia nervosa. *Psychiatric Research, 1,* 209-215.

Hudson, J., Laffer, P., & Pope, H. (1982). Bulimia related to affective disorder by family and response to dexamethasone suppression test. *American Journal of Psychiatry, 139,* 685-687.

Johnson, C., & Flack, R. Family characteristics of bulimic and normal women: A comparative study. Submitted for publication, 1984.

Kalucy, R. S., Crisp, A. H., & Harding, B. (1977). A study of 56 families with anorexia nervosa. *British Journal of Medical Psychiatry, 50,* 381-395.

Keys, A., Brozek, J., Henschel, A., Mickelson, O., & Taylor, H. (1950) *The biology of human starvation.* Minneapolis: University of Minneapolis Press.

Lord, A., & Orleans, C. (1981). Binge eating in obesity: Preliminary findings and guidelines for behavioral analysis and treatment. *Addictive Behaviors, 6,* 155-166.

Minuchin, S., Rosman, B., & Baker, L. (1978). *Psychosomatic families: Anorexia nervosa in context.* Cambridge, Mass.: Harvard University Press.

Norman, D., & Herzog, D. (1983). Bulimia, anorexia nervosa and anorexia nervosa with bulimia: A comparative analysis of MMPI profiles. *International Journal of Eating Disorders, 2,* 43-52.

Nylander, I. (1971). The feeling of being fat and dieting in a school population: Epidemiologic interview investigation. *Acta Sociomedica Scandinavia, 3,* 17-26.

Orbach, S. (1984). Accepting the symptom: A feminist treatment of anorexia nervosa. In D. Garner and P. Garfinkel (Eds.). *Handbook of psychotherapy for anorexia nervosa and bulimia.* New York: Guilford Press.

Pyle, R., Mitchell, J., & Eckert, E. (1981). Bulimia: A report of 34 cases. *Journal of Clinical Psychiatry, 42,* 60-64.

Saleh, J., & Lebwahl, P. (1980). Metoclopramide-induced gastric emptying in patients with anorexia nervosa. *American Jornal of Gastroenterology, 74,* 127-132.

Selvini-Palazzoli, M. (1974). *Anorexia nervosa.* London: Chaucer.

Strober, M. (1981). The significance of bulimia in anorexia nervosa: A multivariate analysis. *Psychosomatic Medicine, 43,* 323-330.

Strober, M. (1983). An empirically derived typology of anorexia nervosa. In P. Darby, P. Garfinkel, D. Garner, and D. Coscina (Eds.). *Anorexia nervosa: Recent developments.* New York: Alan Liss.

Strober, M. (1984). Stressful life events associated with bulimia in anorexia nervosa: Empirical findings and theoretical speculations. *International Journal of Eating Disorders, 3,* 3-16.

Strober, M., Salkin, B., Burroughs, J., & Morrell, W. (1982). Validity of the bulimia-restricter distinction in anorexia nervosa. *Journal of Nervous and Mental Disease, 170,* 345-351.

Vandereycken, W., & Pierloot, R. (1983). Dropout during inpatient treatment of anorexia nervosa: A clinical study of 133 patients. In W. Minsel & W. Herff (Eds.). *Research on psychotherapeutic approaches.* Frankfurt: Peter Lang.

Wardle, J., & Beinart, H. (1981). Binge eating: A theoretical review. *British Journal of Clinical Psychology, 20,* 97-109.

Weiner, H. (1977). *Psychology and human disease.* New York: Elsevier, North Holland, Inc.

Wooley, O., & Wooley, S. (1982). The Beverly Hills eating disorder: The mass marketing of anorexia nervosa (editorial). *International Journal of Eating Disorders, 1,* 57-69.

Yager, J. (1984). Clinical Notes on Anorexia Nervosa. *Bulletin of the Menninger Clinic, 48,* 427-442.

Occupational Therapy for Patients with Eating Disorders

Mary K. Bailey, OTR, FAOTA

ABSTRACT. The role of the occupational therapist and activity therapy programs for patients with eating disorders is described. Evaluation methods are outlined with specific comments related to their implications for patients with diagnoses of anorexia nervosa and bulimia. Rationale for referral to specific activity therapy services is discussed. Group protocols are included. Two case studies demonstrate the utilization of occupational therapy and other activity therapies with an anorectic patient and a bulimic patient.

The Eating Disorder Program at The Sheppard and Enoch Pratt Hospital consists of six beds housed within a 20-bed adult (ages 18-65), intermediate-care (30-90 days), inpatient hall. All patients including those with eating disorders are provided with activity therapy programming which may include: centralized hospital or hall-based groups and individual counseling to which they are referred for specific treatment objectives, leisure skill development groups which patients select themselves for one-month "courses," and open/optional activities in which patients use facilities (ex: gym, pool, hobbies room) with staff or volunteers who assist their experimentation with new media or provide opportunities to engage in familiar leisure activities.

Referred activity therapy groups are selected by a collaborative effort of the patient and the occupational therapist who functions as the representative or liaison between the hall and the activity therapy department. Selection is based on mutual acknowledgement of problems in areas of work, leisure, self-care, or identification and expression of feelings. Cognitive, motor, and social functioning in the aforementioned areas are evaluated in a variety of ways.

Mary K. Bailey is the Chief, Occupational Therapy Section, and Assistant Director, Activity Therapy Department, at The Sheppard and Enoch Pratt Hospital, Baltimore, Maryland.

EVALUATION METHODS

Each patient receives and completes packet of forms. Leisure activities and values are surveyed on self-report forms based on Max Kaplan's theory of need satisfaction through activity participation (Kaplan, 1960; Herbert, 1969; Schwab, 1976). One form poses questions relating to self-perceived need of or value for engagement in leisure pursuits clustered within seven constructs: new and stimulating, familiar and quiet, altruistic, self-improving, externally organized or structured, creative, social. A companion form examines recent history of participation in activities reprsentative of the same seven constructs. Self-perceived strengths and weaknesses in social skills are reported on a self-attitude survey developed by the occupational therapy department at the Dwight David Eisenhower Medical Center at Fort Gordon, Georgia. The leisure and self-attitude surveys are scored numerically by systems developed by their authors. An additional questionnaire requires short narrative statements by the patient in answer to questions regarding stress management and independent living skills: cooking, use of community resources, apartment living, and money management.

All patients participate in a one-hour group session in which they are asked to complete two tasks. One involves the use of paper, pencil, and ruler. Four verbal directions are given before the patients begin. This is a highly structured individual task. Evaluators score (on a scale of 1 to 5) such factors as memory, distractibility, dexterity, problem-solving ability, mental imagery, ability to parallel or generalize. The last two factors are elicited during a short discussion, and the patients are encouraged to consider their own reaction to the process.

The second task involves the creation of a group mural using pastels on a large sheet of brown paper. Evaluators score the following group interaction skills: participation, leadership, assertiveness, and negotiation and compromise in theme choice; participation, awareness of others, support of others, and social exchanges during the drawing.

In the short discussion following completion of the tasks, leaders assess the accuracy of the patients' perceptions of their own and others' roles in the activity. Again, patients are encouraged to examine the differences in their reactions to the individual structured, and the group unstructured experiences. They are advised to discuss preferences, strengths, and problem areas with their activity therapy representatives as treatment schedules are developed.

Patients attend a one-hour session in the gymnasium to evaluate gross motor function. For the first 30 minutes, they are invited to choose among a number of unstructured activities: paddle ball, shooting baskets, badminton, frisbee catch, etc. A team game is organized during the second 30 minutes. Evaluators assess patients' familiarity with sports, coordination, posture, reflexive reaction, flexibility, and pace. Group interaction and team skills are also assessed as well as the patients' approach or reaction to physical competition. Further screening is done for any obvious perceptual difficulties.

Evaluation of gross motor skills is delayed for newly admitted and severely cachetic, anorexia nevosa patients. Even when exercise is medically indicated, evaluators note and limit any tendency to over-exercise in the quest for "burning" calories.

Each patient also participates in a group (four to five people) evaluation/orientation session co-led by a dance therapist and an art therapist. Movement and drawings are evaluated and discussed. The resulting written report forwarded to the occupational therapist also includes recommendations regarding referral to dance and/or art therapy.

The occupational therapist interviews each patient individually (Shaw, 1982). during the 45-60-minute interview, data is gathered regarding the patient's history and status immediately prior to admission in the areas of work or school, living situation, leisure and social pursuits and preferences. Problems, strengths, limitations, and resources are mutually identified using the results of the aforementioned procedures as well as data and opinions offered by the patient. The occupational therapist and the patient establish goals for treatment and discuss resources within the activity therapy program for addressing the identified problems, utilizing identified strengths and preferences and working toward agreed-upon goals.

PROGRAMMING

The occupational therapist is responsible for developing a schedule of activities for each patient. Referrals are written for groups, such as dance therapy, leisure education, cooking, ceramics; and/or for individual counseling, such as vocational counseling, leisure counseling, money management, apartment living. When the schedule of referred activity therapy sesions and individual or group psychotherapy is established, the new patient is counseled by the occupational therapist regarding selection of optional groups from the skill development and open activity schedules. Thus, the patient's first weekly schedule is established (Figure 1). Schedules are regularly reviewed, and progress reports are written twice monthly for the first 90 days and monthly therafter by group leaders and counselors who forward them to the referring occupational therapist. As the patients' needs change, new referrals are written, and schedules are modified accordingly.

ROLE OF THE OCCUPATIONAL THERAPIST

The assessment and programming responsibilities described above are part of the occupational therapist's role as activity therapy representative to the 20-bed hall. Additional components include documentation in the medical charts of all patients, participation in hall (patient and staff) meetings, hall staff meetings (clinical and administrative), patient evaluation and reevaluation conferences. Additional activity therapy staff with part-time resonsibilities to the hall include a dance therapist, an art therapist, a recreation therapist, and a vocational counselor. Coordination of their direct and indirect patient services is a part of the occupational therapist's role.

Additional clinical responsibilities include co-leading with a member of the nursing staff a *New Comer's Group* designed for orientation of all patients new to the hall. It is held twice weekly and touches on such subjects as hospital treatment philosophy, treatment team members, and hall procedures. Leaders facilitate patients' discussion of their fears and fantasies about hopitalization and how they experience the environment in the early days. Each patient attends a total of three sessions in the first and second weeks of hospitalization.

A group held twice weekly to acquaint the new patient with the activity therapy building and programs is co-led with a recreation therapist. This experiential group utilizes a variety of activities and facilities including: the greenhouse, the library, the hobbies room, the leather and ceramics area, the kitchen, and the game room. The group leaders involve other activity therapy staff as indicated in ses-

Name DOE, JANE   WEEKLY SCHEDULE   3/1/85   M.K. BAILEY   X 2308

TIME	SUNDAY	MONDAY	TUESDAY	WEDNESDAY	THURSDAY	FRIDAY	SATURDAY
8:00 - 8:30							
8:30 - 9:00		HALL MTNG.				HALL MTNG.	
9:00 - 9:30							
9:30 - 10:00		PSYCHOTHERAPY	VALUES CLARIFICATION	PSYCHOTHERAPY	VALUES CLARIFICATION	PSYCHOTHERAPY	
10:00 - 10:30		↓	↓	↓	↓	↓	
10:30 - 11:00							
11:00 - 11:30		CERAMICS	DANCE THERAPY	CERAMICS	DANCE THERAPY	LEISURE COUNSELING	
11:30 - 12:00		↓	↓	↓	↓	↓	
12:00 - 12:30							
12:30 - 1:00							
1:00 - 1:30		EATING ANXIETY GROUP	FEELINGS GROUP	ART THERAPY	ASSERTIVE COMMUNICATIONS GROUP	ART THERAPY	
1:30 - 2:00		↓	↓	↓	↓	↓	OPEN HOBBIES
2:00 - 2:30	OPEN SWIM		↓	↓	↓	↓	
2:30 - 3:00							↓
3:00 - 3:30	↓	NATURE HIKE		HALL MTNG.		NATURE HIKE	
3:30 - 4:00		↓	VOCATIONAL COUNSELING	↓		↓	
4:00 - 4:30		↓	↓		EATING ANXIETY GROUP	FEELINGS GROUP	
4:30 - 5:00					↓	↓	
5:00 - 5:30							
5:30 - 6:00							
6:00 - 6:30			TRANSITIONS GROUP				
6:30 - 7:00			↓	HALL TRIP			
7:00 - 7:30	MOVIE (7-9)		HALL MTNG.	↓	HALL MTNG.		

Form 118 270 R384   ※ REFERRED A.T. SERVICES   THE SHEPPARD AND ENOCH PRATT HOSPITAL

FIGURE 1

93

sions which move from one area to another, some of which are held outdoors. At the end of each group hour, the activity is discussed by patients and staff in terms of its potential for therapeutic application. Each patient attends six to eight sessions.

The patients involved in the Eating Disorder Program have a number of ongoing hall-based treatment activities included as a part of the established protocol (see article by David Roth, Ph.D, in this issue). Of these, the occupational therapist is involved in one, the *Assertive Communications Group,* co-led by the occupational therapist and a member of the hall's nursing staff. While patients in the eating disorder program are required to attend, the group members include other patients who reside on their hall.

CLINICAL IMPLICATIONS: PATIENTS WITH EATING DISORDERS

Evaluation. The descriptions and dynamics of anorexia nervosa and bulimia patients are contained in other sections of this issue. In the activity therapy program, some significant patterns have emerged in evaluation procedures. Anorexia nervosa patients demonstrate little awareness of their own needs/values as measured in the leisure survey forms. Similarly, reported frequency in the related activities is far lower than is normal for women in their age group. By contrast, bulimic women often report investment in need identification as well as practice in one area of leisure activity with depressed scores for all others. It seems that they often pick one construct or area (for example, "sociability") in which to invest their energies to the exclusion of all others.

Almost without exception, women with eating disorders report dramatically lowered self-esteem with scores on the self-attitude survey lower even than those of other women with identified psychiatric disorders.

Anorectic and bulimic patients are clearly more comfortable with the very structured task described earlier as a part of the evaluation process. Their perfectionistic (Stober, 1980) tendencies lend themselves to tasks with predetermined end results, so their "perfection" is clearly recognizable. Their group interaction skills are uniformly diminished despite high level verbal and cognitive functioning, and they seem reluctant to involve themselves in a task in which they cannot control the outcome.

In the dance and art therapy assessments, body image distortions, painful self-consciousness, fear of expressive movement, sense of disconnected body parts, and immature images are among the usual reported findings (Bruch, 1982).

PROGRAMMING IN ACTIVITY THERAPY

An *Assertive Communications Group* (Appendix A) (Alberti, 1974; Smith, 1975; Galassi, 1977) is included regularly in the schedule of the eating disorder patient. The basic concepts of the group address the self-esteem and control issues evident in women with eating disorders. Identification and appropriate expression of feelings in relationships are problematic for the anorectic woman who experiences only a narrow range of emotional reactions and who senses that, in any event, her feelings don't count (Bruch, 1982). As she begins to become aware of her emotions in psychotherapy, dance therapy, art therapy, and milieu groups, it is helpful to explore techniques for expression as well as to experience the curative factor of "universality" described by Yalom (1975). The anorectic woman discovers that others are sharing the pain of emerging awareness and the frustration of attempting to express feelings in a mature and effective way.

Of particular importance is anticipating and rehearsing (role playing) assertive ways to address changes in family relationships. Family therapy is a dynamic component of the total treatment program. The Assertive Communications Group provides patients with a supportive environment in which to examine and validate, review and rehearse their attempts at establishing independent and adult membership in the family group. Indeed, one of the technical problems the group co-leaders face is structuring sessions so that members learn to "walk before they run." It is important to remember that practicing assertive techniques in less emotionally loaded situations will assist in the integration of the concepts of assertive communication and will perhaps ease their use in the more critical areas of life. Thus, we use hall meetings, roommate differences, and hypothetical situations to begin the learning process.

Some centralized (all hospital) occupational therapy groups utilize specific objectives for patients with eating disorders. *The Cooking Group* (Appendix B) is often useful, and although it is designed primarily as an ADL group, expectations and goals for treatment are modified for the anorectic or bulimic patients. These young women usually have a far better than average knowledge of caloric content of foods, but they need information regarding other basic food content. The experience of cooking and eating normal size portions is useful for women who have demonstrated idiosyncratic cooking and eating habits.

The *Ceramics Group* (Appendix C) has been valuable for a variety of reasons. Starting with slipcasting with a predetermined and fairly controllable outcome, patients are later encouraged to experiment with slab and coil construction and use of the potter's wheel. Initially, they experience real pain when self-perceived flaws occur in their pieces. With support and validation from group members and leaders, they learn to experiment and to appreciate artistic imperfections. This ability to relinquish perfectionistic control and to experience pride and pleasure in completion of a piece that looks handmade rather than slick and manufactured is often a sign of progress. If the connection can be made to other areas of the patient's life, an important self-esteem issue has been addressed.

The *Leatherwork Group* (Appendix D), as with the ceramics group, provides a useful third-object activity for patients with eating disorders. Using this more controllable medium, the initial anxiety is perhaps less. However, self-expectations of the confirmed perfectionist are often sadly thwarted when she finds she cannot immediately master complex tools and processes. She learns she must establish realistic short-term goals and begin to take pride in each day's achievement as opposed to experiencing defeat and frustration when unable to function as a master craftsman. The group leader encourages and facilitates the patient's ability to identify for herself those components of the project that may be realistically completed in one or two sessions. Again, if the lesson learned is generalized to other areas of life, the establishment and accomplishment of short-term goals can address control and self-esteem issues. Leather is a particularly useful medium as progress is easily discerned in both tool mastery and project complexity.

Other activity therapy groups to which eating disorder patients are frequently referred may include *Weight Training Group*, where the patient can learn that she can control her exercise appropriately rather than be a slave to it (Garfinkel, 1982). *Dance Therapy* may help to promote positive bodily perceptions (Garfinkel, 1982) as well as to assist the patient in a growing awareness of her emotional reactions and needs as experienced in bodily sensations and movement. In *Art Therapy*, patients' progress is monitored by examining the integration of body images, use of color and line, maturity of figures and content (Murphy, 1983). Young women are often involved in educational and vocational decisions and pursuits. Scholastic achievement is an area where psychopathology is demonstrated (Garfinkel, 1982), and *Vocational Counseling* may be of practical value in the establishment of realistic scholastic and career goals. A *Transitions Group,* led by a recreation therapist, helps patients to consider previously dysfunctional leisure patterns and to explore community resources and supports. Social out-of-hospital visits to various Baltimore area museums, theaters, and support groups are encouraged. Dining in area restaurants is often recommended just before discharge for patients with eating disorders.

CASE STUDIES

1. Barbara is a nineteen-year-old, unmarried, freshman college student admitted to The Sheppard and Enoch Pratt Hospital's eating disorder program in the spring of 1984. At 5'2'', she weighed 78 pounds at the time of admission. She reported symptoms of mood variability, fatigue, impaired concentration, hypotension, hypothermia, and amenorrhea. She demonstrated typically anorectic eating habits, such as cutting up foods into extremely small pieces, taking inordinately long periods of time to complete a meal, avoiding "dangerous" fattening foods like butter, salad dressings, etc. She reported daily routines of excessive exercising which had largely replaced previously enjoyed leisure activities, such as playing piano, painting, and volunteer work with children in day care centers and summer camps.

The third of four children, Barbara has an older brother and two sisters, one older and one younger. Her parents are both professional people, intelligent and articulate. At Barbara's admission, her mother was tearful, intensely concerned about the details of her daughter's anticipated care, especially medical monitoring. She disclosed details of a disturbed family constellation including her own and her husband's "chronic characterologic depressions." Barbara's brother had received treatment for depression. Both mother and older sister experienced brief periods of anorexia in the past. Various individual and family therapies have been a part of the family's life for some years. Barbara saw herself as a mediator between mother and father.

Barbara was overweight during high school years at approximately 140 pounds and attributed feelings of social isolation and rejection to her weight. She began dieting and by the time she entered college weighed 100 pounds. Her first experience of living away from home was traumatic and involved tearful phone calls home and anxiety attacks. She terminated that attempt at college by Christmas of 1982 and began outpatient therapy after returning to live at home. She entered college again in the fall of 1983 and was able to continue college and live away from home until the time of admission. Throughout the 18 months from fall of 1982 until spring of 1984, she struggled with anorexia despite outpatient therapy. Her admission to hospital was at the urgent recommendation of her therapist when her weight loss and vital signs became a source of alarm.

Barbara had always been an achiever. An "A" student, she also excelled at the studio arts, modern dance, and violin. Her perfectionistic standards were evident in the activity therapy evaluation. She was acutely uncomfortable during the art and dance therapy evaluation process despite familiarity with both media. Her picture was childlike in content, use of color, and poorly defined human figures. Her movement was constricted and protective. The overall score on her self-attitude survey was low with self-perceived problems in establishing and maintaining relationships with others. Her leisure surveys reflected her recent history of denial of needs and restriction of activity other than excessive exercise.

In the initial occupational therapy interview, Barbara sat quietly with folded hands in a "good child" posture. She spoke in a soft but audible voice, describing her situation clearly and articulately. She professed to be eagerly anticipating involvement in the activity therapy program as soon as she was permitted to leave the hall (see Eating Disorder Program Protocol described by David Roth, Ph.D., in this issue). She indicated that she was continuing her college studies while in the hospital and would need to arrange a schedule which would include study time. Though Barbara described an extensive repertoire of leisure and social pursuits and skills, two distinct patterns seemed evident. She had discontinued all leisure activities except running and swimming laps. Though she stated she had many friends and had been involved in social activities with groups and with individual young women friends, she had never dated. She agreed with the evaluator's assessment of her perfectionistic drive for superachievement and found the notion that she might work on that in a ceramics group to be intriguing. She was able to acknowledge that her view of her body was apparently distorted. The interviewer saw this self-assessment as an attempt at compliance rather than a truly integrated insight. Barbara saw referral to dance and art therapies as an opportunity to address this problem, as well as to explore and develop awareness of feelings. The fact that she had familiarity with both media eased the doubts and fears usually expressed by anorectic women. A water therapy referral was agreed upon as a compromise between the contraindicated vigorous exercise groups she proposed and a schedule of sedentary activites. (Lap swimming is not included in the water therapy protocol.) Barbara had made no career goals or decisions at that point, and though there was certainly no immediate pressure to do this, she indicated an interest in utilizing the services of a hospital vocational counselor to explore aptitudes, interests, and various options for the future. Barbara indicated an awareness of her own passive and indirect style of communicating needs and feelings, problems she would address in the assertive communications group.

Although the initial interview appeared to be mutually productive, the interviewer was aware of the patient's need to be seen as "good" and speculated that her willingness to share problems and to participate in exploring resources to address them was not necessarily a predictor of investment over time. Barbara had perfect attendance to her activity therapy groups despite some early struggles. In ceramics, she was unable at first to work on more than one project at a time despite waiting periods at various stages in her pieces. She was distressed to find a small chip in a mold and said she "would never have used it" had she known. She was unable to experiment and needed much guidance from the group leader. She related singularly to the group leader and isolated herself from others in the group during sessions.

In art therapy, Barbara struggled to create perfect pictures during the first few sessions. Her productions were detailed, precise, and overcontrolled. Self-representational images were fractured, and overall themes were childlike. In assertive communications, Barbara seemed to assume an intellectual "clarifier" role. She clearly understood concepts and worked to comply in role plays and exercises. Her overall demeanor was stiff, overcontrolled, lacking in spontaneity. Although she was able to share self-perceived difficulties with various assertive behaviors, she demonstrated little ability to modify her habitual passive and self-effacing manner during early sessions.

Water therapy group leaders noted special need for monitoring Barbara's drive to overexercise, especially at the beginning and ending of each session. This remained a difficulty throughout her hospitalization in activity therapy groups, open activities, and while on trips and visits outside the hospital. Various contracts and contingency arrangements were only marginally successful in assisting her in overcoming her bondage to calorie-burning exercise.

Within six weeks, Barbara was able to work on two or three ceramic pieces at once and to work more independently with less attention to precise detail. She tried some experimentation with evident discomfort yet felt pride in her ability to loosen up a bit. In art therapy, her pictures were somewhat more free in graphic expression and became reflective of her internal control vs freedom conflicts. In assertive communications, Barbara began to rehearse interactions with her family, particularly her mother. She was able to cry in the group when disclosing her mother's ability to predict her "failures" and her consequent loss of confidence and her inability to defend her own positions. The group discussed various assertive approaches and supported her early, awkward attempts at individuation. She received validation and applause on the few occasions that she was able to effect a specific change in her own behavior, apparently influencing a change in her mother's behavior.

In dance therapy, issues of independence, direct expression of angry feelings and integration of movement and feelings were addressed. Barbara never achieved flowing spontaneous movement but apparently gained awareness of the bodily sensations associated with various feeling states.

Determination of a specific career objective had not been a treatment goal although Barbara used vocational counseling and testing to narrow her focus somewhat to art or education or a combination thereof.

At time of discharge, Barbara had met or paritally met most of her treatment goals. She achieved goal weight (105 pounds) and sustained it for one month before discharge. She recognized and had been able to relinquish many of her perfectionistic habits. Still oriented to achievement, she could at least consider the possibility of earning something less than "straight A's" in school. This was accompanied by an acknowledgment of needed and valued leisure activities not involving competition with self-determined and unrealistic goals or with other people seen as ideal role models. Newly acquired assertiveness was demonstrated in the context of confrontive and supportive remarks offered in hall meetings although Barbara never achieved the voice volume and assertive body posture she and her treatment team might have wished. She had a very clear idea of the quality of the relationship she wanted to attain with her mother and had integrated a few attitudes and techniques toward that end. Her art therapy productions were reflective of newly formed awareness of feeling states and continued to show improving and more mature self-perceptions. She was discharged to return to school with plans to continue in group therapy with other eating disorder patients, individual therapy, and family therapy.

2. Christine is a 22-year-old, single, white, graduate student admitted to the eating disorder unit during the winter of 1983-84. She was a self-referral who reported a six-year history of bulimia which she felt had been "out of control" in the six weeks before admission. Additionally, she indicated she had been depressed in varying degrees since approximately age six. She had been involved in outpatient therapy during her college career, utilizing time-limited groups within which she had acknowledged her depression but withheld information about her bulimia. At time of admission, she was slender but not wasted. In fact, she was attractive and at near-normal weight.

Christine was the second of four children with an older brother and two younger sisters. Her brother received psychiatric treatment as a youngster, a short time after his father's death. Christine's early memories of her father included his protracted and debilitating illness, visits to hospitals, and his death when she was eight. Her mother was employed as a teacher and was apparently self-sufficient. Both mother and daughter described a mutually supportive, sometimes difficult, and certainly enmeshed relationship. Christine indicated that she felt that she was the closest of the children to her mother though they had not actually lived together since she started college. During Christine's early years, her mother was unavailable to her much of the time, as she was preoccupied with caring for her husband until his death and was subsequently concerned about Christine's brother's emotional problems.

Always a good student, Christine graduated from a private college preparatory school and attended a prestigious "ivy league" university for undergraduate studies. As a part of her school work and in extracurricular studies, she became an accomplished dancer. During summer vacations and part time during the school year, she worked as a dancer. She also had several temporary and part-time jobs as a model, sales clerk, and waitress, experiencing occasional difficulty accepting supervision from those she felt to be her intellectual inferiors.

Superficially social and friendly, Christine reported that she routinely dealt with stress by isolating herself, trying to alleviate her depression by planning changes in her environment and/or life goals, and ultimately eating and vomiting to relieve anxiety and worry.

Christine's intelligence and perfectionism were evident in her completion of the structured task in her activity therapy evaluation. She participated actively and effectively in the group task but indicated a preference for working alone whether involved in structured or unstructured tasks. In the leisure self-report forms, her denial of need for leisure satisfaction was evident except within the construct reflective of self-improvement activities (courses, museum visits, etc.). She indicated a recent and marked decline in the frequency of her participation in all leisure activities, particularly those strictly social in nature. In the self-attitude survey, Christine indicated low self-esteem, and a passive-aggressive coping style was revealed in the pattern of her responses.

In the art and dance therapy evaluation session, Christine reflected despair in slow movement, bent posture, and use of dark, dismal colors and content in her picture. During the initial occupational therapy interview, Christine wept frequently. Tears seemed to appear and flow even when her voice and facial expression did not seem particularly sad. She spoke of her life in recent months as being an unsatisfying combination of school drudgery and endless meetings of Overeaters Anonymous and Alcoholics Anonymous. In following OA guidelines, she was obliged to weigh all her food meticulously and eat specific types of food. She stated that following these guidelines precluded any spontaneous social life, especially those activities which might include eating or taking place where food might be available. Her attendance at AA meetings was not because of a drinking problem but was an attempt at using AA concepts and guidelines for conquering her binging and purging. About six weeks before admission, she decided that her life had no joy or meaning, so she stopped attending meetings and began a month of "out-of-control" binging, purging, and sometimes restricting. She described that period of time as "nightmarish."

She indicated that even before her eating disorder had become so intrusive, her leisure was rarely designed for enjoyment but had centered around those activities she saw as "important," such as the arts, museums, lectures, and music. She stated that she experienced disappointment and frustration early in life when she perceived others as critical and rejecting, so she rarely looked to other people for support. Through the years, she had two good women friends and two intimate relationships with men. The first heterosexual relationship was terminated when he was killed in an accident. The second had been problematic for about two years at the time of admission, compromised by her secretive eating habits and his anger and confusion. Clearly, his presence in her life was a complication, not a support.

Christine appeared to be open and spontaneous during interview, but she was dubious about utilizing activity therapy services to address acknowledged and mutually agreed-upon problems. She was aware of and described her defense of "intellectualizing" to avoid feelings and agreed to try nonverbal art and dance therapies to assist her in identifying feeling states through movement and imagery. Interestingly, an appeal to her intellect by sharing group protocols was useful in enlisting her participation. She was intrigued with the notion of utilizing values clarification exercises in an effort to explore her own beliefs and preferences in a structured group environment. She was interested in learning about ceramics and agreed to "work on" her strivings for perfection within this medium. Her attendance in assertive communications group was assured by the protocol of the eating disorder program. She described her own style of relating as passive although evaluation and assessment procedures and observation had persuaded all members of her treatment team that she was most often aggressive or passive-aggressive in stressful encounters with others.

Christine began activity therapy groups with initial bravado and a rather flamboyant aura of superiority. She seemed charismatic to other group members, assumed leadership roles, demonstrated a dry and sometimes cutting wit. As she became engaged in the processes, a number of different behaviors were exhibited. In art therapy, pictures were dark, dismal, and she spoke openly of her depressed feelings and general sense of hopelessness. In dance therapy, she struggled with a relationship with another group member who reminded her of her younger sister with whom she was alternately overprotective and rejecting. She was never able to work effectively within the dance therapy group, always working apart, as though in an individual session. Her movements were sometimes aggressive, somewhat frenetic, and sometimes slow, bent, and despairing. Always dramatic, she elicited a variety of reactions from group members ranging from awed admiration to hostility and jealousy.

In early sessions of the assertive communications group, Christine appeared to doze. In later weeks, she was able to identify this as a symptom of her anxiety. She perceived herself as passive in interactions with others, yet group members quickly began to identify her controlled, rational, sometimes sarcastic demeanor as aggressive or passive-aggressive. Confronted by their feedback, she seemed initially bewildered. Slowly, she was able to relinquish her superficial air of bored superiority and began to demonstrate a desire to emphasize the communications aspect of the group to improve her ability to form relationships, to give and receive support. She brought instances of interactions with others which she had found confusing to the group. For example, part of her program included involvement in a hospitalwide patient committee which functions to provide evening and weekend social events. Committee membership is voluntary, and each officer is voted in by incumbent members of the executive committee. Christine achieved the necessary votes, but she was given direct and specific feedback regarding changes the executive committee anticipated in her occasionally intimidating manner. She reported this to the Assertive Communications Group and seemed appreciative of feedback and suggestions, role-playing alternative interaction styles. She functioned as hall chairman (leading hall meetings) for a time and asked for and received interactions with her mother as family therapy and visits home became increasingly important.

From time to time during the course of her hospitalization, Christine became anxious, despondent, fearful of her ability to handle her increasing sensitivity to others after discharge, without falling back on binging-purging behaviors. During those times, she was comforted and supported by the structure present in her Values Clarification Group and Ceramics Group. In both activities, group leaders reported consistent attendance, focus on task and active participation. This was in sharp contrast to her behavior on her hall which was characterized alternately by withdrawal or push of speech, weeping, feeling like a "zombie." She was able to identify activities and structure which apparently provided some alleviation of her distress and spoke in the Transitions Group of beginning to explore community resources for leisure activities which could be utilized in a like fashion.

Vocational counseling sessions resulted in Christine's development of a resume and assistance in job hunting when she had made the decision to delay returning to graduate school and to live and work for a time in the Baltimore area. Before finalizing plans, she participated in a work therapy assignment to focus on work habits in a structured situation and to assess her ability to receive supervision. She was pleased with the respect she earned from co-workers and the success with which she related to them and to supervisors.

Christine continued art theapy until discharge. Her pictures varied dramatically from one session to another. Sometimes, a lightening of mood and sense of optimism was evident. Fear and depression continued in some pictures. Internal chaos seemed threatening and overwhelming as she anticipated discharge. Her recognition and expression of those feelings was significant in that she was learning to seek support from others rather than utilizing old pattens of flight, withdrawal, binging, and purging.

Before discharge, Christine asked for and received referral to the cooking group. She felt she needed opportunities to cook and eat "feared" or "binge" foods. Initially, she had some difficulty accepting group decisions regarding menus, as her own eating habits had been so idiosyncratic and overcontrolled in the recent past. However by the time of discharge, she seemed able to participate as a full group member despite anxieties privately disclosed to the group leader.

For three to four weeks before discharge, Christine began working in a local department store. She had a variety of trips outside the hospital using community resources for social and self-help support groups. She visited local restaurants with other patients and attended events where food was available. All of these ventures were anxiety provoking, but she was able to ask for and receive support from staff and other patients with a repertoire of newly learned, and apparently integrated interpersonal skills. She was discharged with plans to share an apartment with another young woman, work, attend family therapy, individual psychotherapy, and group therapy for people with eating disorders.

FINAL COMMENT

Eating disorders are life threatening. Admission to hospital occurs when patients and their families have become desperate. Pathological defenses and coping styles have become entrenched. Body image distortions have an almost delusional quality. If a treatment program is to be effective, all component parts must be integrated. The occupational therapist must share responsibility with the psychotherapist, social worker, and nursing staff for identifying problems and determining treatment objectives. Ongoing communication among treatment team members is critical, as each uses his own modality for facilitating changes in the patient's self-assessment, interpersonal skills, problem-solving techniques, and life-style. The preceding description of the role of occupational therapy should be understood as occurring within a setting where all members of the treatment team have a common understanding of specific objectives and regularly share information regarding progress toward attaining those objectives throughout each patient's hospital stay.

REFERENCES

Alberti, R., Emmons, M. (1974). *Your Perfect Right*. San Luis Obispo, CA. IMPACT.

Bruch, H. (1982). Anorexia Nervosa: Therapy and Theory. *American Journal of Psychiatry. 139:12*. 1531-1538.

Galassi, Galassi (1979) Assert Yourself! How to be *Your Own Person*. New York: Human Sciences Press.

Garfinkel, P., Garner, D. (1982). *Anorexia Nervosa a Multidimensional Perspective*. New York: Brunner Mazel.

Herbert, E. (1969). *Leisure Interest Inventory*, Doctoral Dissertation, University of North Carolina, Chapel Hill.

Kaplan, M. (1960). *Leisure in America: A Social Inquiry*, Willy.

Mosey, A. (1970). *Three Frames of Reference for Mental Health*, Thorofare, NJ, Charles B. Slack, Inc.

Murphy, P. (1983). *A Study of Art Productions of Persons with Eating Disorders*. Thesis for Master of Arts, Goucher College, Towson, MD.

Schwab, J. (1976). Leisure Counseling: A Counseling Approach Towards the Effective Use of Leisure Time, *Pennsylvania Recreation and Parks*, November, 10-11.

Shaw, C. (1982). The Interview Process. Hemphill, B. (ed.), *The Evaluative Process in Psychiatric Occupational Therapy*, Thorofare, NJ, Slack, Inc.

Smith (1975). *When I Say No, I Feel Guilty*. New York, Dial Press.

Strober, M. (1980). Personality and Symptomatological Features in Young, Nonchronic Anorexia Nervosa Patients. *Journal of Psychosomatic Research, 24*, 353-359.

Yalom, I. (1975). *The Theory and Practice of Group Psychotherapy*. New York: Basic Books, Inc.

APPENDIX A
THE SHEPPARD AND ENOCH PRATT HOSPITAL
ACTIVITY THERAPY DEPARTMENT
ASSERTIVE COMMUNICATIONS GROUP

I. Format:

Time: Thursday 1:15-2:30
Place: A4/A5 Conference Room
Size: 6-8 patients
Leaders: OTR/L
          R.N.

II. Purpose:

The Assertive Communications group was formed and the content developed on the assumption that patients in a state of psychosocial dysfunction frequently experience fear, shame, and guilt with the associated decrease in self-esteem and increase in anxiety surrounding interpersonal relationships and interactions. Using a behavioral frame of reference, the group focuses on common everyday situations (example: making and refusing requests, dealing with criticism). Patients examine basic interpersonal rights (example: the right to say no, the right to privacy, the right to feel and express anger) and the components and consequences of nonassertive, aggressive, and assertive behaviors in situations where those rights are at stake. Opportunities are provided for patients to explore and practice communication techniques and methods of coping with the conflicts in everyday living to decrease anxiety and improve self-confidence.

III. Goals/Behavioral Objectives:

A. Increase Self-Esteem
   Patient will: demonstrate awareness of own interpersonal rights; state opinions convincingly and disagree with aggression.
B. Decrease Anxiety
   Patient will demonstrate: sustained eye contact, absence of nonproductive behaviors (rocking, playing with hands, etc.),

an audible tone of voice comfortably erect posture, emphatic gestures, meaningful facial expression, spontaneity and flexibility in expression of self.

C. Develop Verbal Communication Ability

Patient will acknowledge that he/she is comfortable carrying on conversations, expressing feelings and opinions.

D. Develop Appropriately Assertive Behavior

Patient will be able to stand up for his interpersonal rights; will act in own best interest without infringing on the rights of others.

IV. Criteria for Patient Referral:

A. The patient should be assigned to hall A5.
B. The patient should demonstrate a willingness to participate.
C. Patients referred to this group should be able to participate in the cooperative group level (Mosey, 1970):

1. Has all day attention span
2. Can think through cause and effect relationships
3. Can establish own goals
4. Can conceive end result
5. Can think through alternatives via covert imagery
6. Can follow three or more written or verbal directions

D. Patient should show potential to become more verbally expressive.

V. Method of Referral:

The A5 patient may be referred by members of his/her treatment team during A5 service conferences. One of the co-leaders will interview the referred patient to ascertain his/her wilingness and apparent ability to participate in and benefit from the group.

VI. Methodology:

The group will operate as a discussion group and will use role play for practice of specific communication techniques.

VII. Leadership:

A. Role of leaders

1. Provide verbal and written orientation to and instruction in concepts of assertiveness and specific communication techniques
2. Offer and promote behavioral feedback
3. Provide role-play situations and facilitate group members supplying personal situations for group discussion and role-play
4. Act as role models for assertive behavior and clear communications

B. Qualification of Leaders
Co-leadership is interdisciplinary. Qualifications are reviewed regarding academic training or a training program that meets the practice standards of the discipline at Sheppard Pratt. One co-leader will be experienced with demonstrated proficiency and will provide support and supervision for the less experienced leader.

VIII. Supervision:

Provided by Service Chief A5, or his designee.

APPENDIX B
THE SHEPPARD AND ENOCH PRATT HOSPITAL
ACTIVITY THERAPY DEPARTMENT
LIFESKILLS PROGRAM: COOKING SKILLS LAB

I. General Information:

Time: Wednesday 12-2:30 p.m.
Place: A.T. Kitchen, Room 16
Size: 5-8 participants
Coach: OTR

II. Description:

In this Learning Lab segment of the Lifeskills Program, participants will actively plan a variety of menus, prepare and sample the dishes, and concretize the total learning experience through discussion of the task skills involved as well as related topics (see Section V). Each activity, whether occurring in the Lab or in the community (supermarket shopping), will be selected for its applicability to the participants' definite or probable discharge plans.

III. Learning Objectives:

The participant will:

1. a. recognize and perform a fair share of the meal preparation during each session . . . or
   b. independently or with some coaching prepare a specific item of his/her own selection.
2. appropriately use kitchen tools/utensils/appliances and materials and will demonstrate understanding of various cooking methods.
3. be active in either group or individual planning, problem solving, decision-making related to the Cooking Lab activities.
4. demonstrate awareness of related skills, such as reading a recipe, measuring ingredients correctly, timing cooking correctly, safety factors, eliminating potential hazards in the kitchen, food costs, and budgeting.
5. the participant's menu choices will be based on a balance between his/her personal food preferences, preferences of others sharing the meal, and acceptable nutritional needs.
6. give evidence of some personally held values regarding the nutritional and social aspects of eating/dining (i.e., "junk food," overeating, dieting).
7. collaborate with the Lab Coach in evaluating his/her level of skills and need for further lab practice.

IV. Criteria for Cooking Lab Referrals:

Patients who are appropriate will demonstrate at least egocentric-cooperative group skills and understand the desirability of having a moderate level of cooking skill. They will be able to follow step-by-step instructions without/with a minimal degree of coaching and be willing to see a task through to completion.

Individuals with physical problems which interfere with normal alimentation will be individually evaluated for appropriateness (gastrointestinal problems, gall bladder, hypoglycemia, diabetes, obesity, anorexia, etc.).

V. Topics Addressed:

Though the principal focus will be increasing the participant's cooking skills, attention will also be directed to related topics/skills, such as:

—Supermarket know how
—How to use leftovers
—Storing food
—Health and safety factors
—Setting an inviting table
—Small scale entertaining
—Social Skills related to dining
—Decision-making, problem solving, and values awareness directly related to meal preparation.

VI. Role of Lab Coach:

—Clarifies the learning objectives
—Guides and facilitates the participion of each group member
—Assesses each individual's level of skill development
—Has major responsibility for health and safety factors
—Actively promotes the related skills referred to in Section V
—Reports directly to the A.T. Representative through the designated evaluation method

VII. Evaluation Method:

A written checklist will be discussed with each referred patient prior to beginning the Cooking Skills Lab. The coach will assist the participant to reassess his/her learning following each lab session and the checklist updated accordingly. A joint decision will be made as to when the participant has reached a level of mastery appropriate for his/her discharge plans.

APPENDIX C
THE SHEPPARD AND ENOCH PRATT HOSPITAL ACTIVITY THERAPY DEPARTMENT CERAMICS PROTOCOL

I. Format:

Group: Ceramics
Time: Monday/Wednesday 11-12
Place: Room 3
Size: 6-8 patients
Leaders: OTR

II. Purpose:

The purposes of this group are broad. Focus areas include cognitive, interpersonal, and psychological development as well as growth in task performance and leisure skills. The primary emphasis of the group will vary depending on the individual patient's need and level of functioning.

III. Goals and Objectives:

A. Improve cognitive/task performance as demonstrated by the ability to:

—follow two-step oral directions
—choose project/methodology which is reasonable in terms of time, skill, and complexity
—set an appropriate pace in relation to task
—attend sessions regularly and punctually
—concentrate on task for at least 45 minutes
—accept supervision and instruction from leader

B. Improve interpersonal skills by demonstrating ability to:

—cooperate with others regarding cleanup and sharing of tools and space

—compromise and negotiate in a manner which is neither overly compliant nor aggressive
—respect others opinions and feelings
—give and seek assistance

C. Improve psychological awareness and comfort by demonstrating ability to:

—accurately perceive own and others' feelings
—express satisfaction regarding quality and investment in project
—express pleasure/pride in achievement regarding completion of project
—express pleasure regarding the creative experience.

D. Improve leisure task/social skills by demonstrating ability to:

—utilize available resources with minimal assistance from group leader
—recognize need and value of ceramics as a potential post-discharge leisure activity

IV. Criteria for Patient Referral:

A. Able to participate in individual activities which require some interaction, sharing, and cooperation.
B. Able to attend to task for at least 45 minutes.
C. Able to follow two oral and one written direction.

V. Methodology:

Patients will be instructed in basic ceramic techniques, including slipcasting, slab and coil construction, and potters wheel. The construction technique, the teaching methods, and the relationship with the leader will be varied and graded to meet the functional level of the patient.

As patients are able, they will be encouraged to participate in group interaction through cooperative patient teaching and assistance, joint cleanup, sharing of tools, and mutual discussion.

The role of leader is to instruct, to set appropriate task and behavioral limits, to give accurate performance feedback, and to explain treatment goals. The leader also supports patients, encourages independence and social interaction, and assists patients in developing a sense of mastery and creativity.

VI. Evaluation:

Patients will be evaluated regarding the frequency of their observed demonstration of the specific objectives.

Exit criteria from the group will involve patients meeting appropriately three-quarters of the objectives on a frequent basis. Recommendations to other groups will be made based on observations of a remaining specific deficit.

APPENDIX D
THE SHEPPARD AND ENOCH PRATT HOSPITAL
ACTIVITY THERAPY DEPARTMENT
LEATHERWORK PROTOCOL

I. Format:

Times:	Monday, Wednesday, 10-11 a.m.
Group Leader:	OTR
Place:	Room 03, Ground Floor, Activities Building
Size:	6-8 patients per group

II. Purpose:

Utilizing leather as a craft modality, the group is designed to provide therapeutically selected and modified activities to meet particular and specific needs of the individual patient with psychosocial dysfunction. The primary focus is on the cognitive processes involved in task performance. The activities are continually graded to meet patient goals and needs.

III. Goals/Objectives:

The following is a list of some of the objectives which may be achieved. The patient will frequently:

1. make decisions concerning the selection of tasks, tools, and methods; consulting with staff for goal-related appropriateness and for needed assistance.
2. carry out relatively complex (occasionally demonstrated) two to three oral and one to two written directions.
3. identify and solve problems which arise in the performance of an acitivity; utilizing resources in an appropriate manner.
4. work on tasks for 75 percent of each session without being distracted by extraneous noise and movement or needing nontask-related breaks.
5. within the structure of the group, utilize the leather process to express hostility, compulsiveness, etc. (i.e., pounding, repetition), seldom expressing these feelings and tendencies in a nonconstructive manner.
6. demonstrate improved self-esteem through increased investment, successful project completion, improved affect, and increased expression of satisfaction about his/her work and him/herself, and willingness to attempt more complex tasks.
7. indicate an increased awareness of others needs and/or feelings by not ignoring them or making depreciatory comments, by honoring reasonable requests, and by giving positive and negative feedback in an empathetic, constructive manner.
8. manipulate tools and materials successfully, thus demonstrating an improvement in manual dexterity and eye-hand coordination.
  _____ and on a most-of-the-time basis:
9. demonstrate the ability to perform tasks of gradually increased complexity, required independence and duration.
10. prior to beginning a project, plan the task and be able to describe the general finished appearance and the approximate, realistic time that will be required for completion.
11. cooperate with others in sharing tools and supplies, assuming appropriate responsibility for clean-up, giving and seeking assistance, following directions, and trying out reasonable suggestions.

IV. Criteria:

Patients referred to the group should generally be able to participate in an upper parallel to project level activity: (Mosey, 1970)

1. Able to cooperate in task, group, and with staff 50 percent of the time.
2. Able to exemplify independent behavior 25 percent of the time.
3. Able to participate in individual activities which require some interaction, sharing, and cooperation.
4. Able to follow at least two oral, one written direction.
5. Minimum attention span of 15-20 minutes.
6. Able to organize simple activities with minimal frustration.
7. Able to remember instructions 40-50 percent of the time.
8. Able to manipulate tools and materials with some assistance.

V. Leadership and Approach:

Group leader will:

1. provide gradation of activities (from simple project or methods to more complex ones) in relation to specific patient needs.
2. reinforce appropriate interactional behavior.
3. encourage "trial and error" experiences and provide opportunities to try again in case of error.
4. explain treatment goals to patient and give performance feedback.

VI. Evaluation—Leatherwork Performance Evaluation

Characteristics and Treatment
of Families with Anorectic Offspring

Nancy Alexander, MSW, LCSW, ACSW

ABSTRACT. Four major theorists specializing in anorexia nervosa were reviewed, and a collective set of family characteristics was developed. Three families, their dynamics, and treatment are then described and compared to the "Theoretical Standard." The greatest area of commonality between the three families was found to be in the area of problematic communication.

PREFACE

Although anorexia nervosa has been a recognized disease entity since the 1800's, the attention of the psychiatric community has been riveted on this tragic and compelling disorder in recent years due to increased incidence.

Attention has turned to the families so clearly poised, with their children, on the brink of disaster. After discussion and publication of the earlier findings, it became clear that there were indeed some distinct features in these families. Although theorists from divergent backgrounds and philosophies approached the problem differently, there were areas of high correlation in their findings. These differences affect the way that treatment is approached and conducted, but when trying to *define, describe,* or *identify* these families, the theoretical differences may in fact be reduced to a difference in perspective on the issue of circularity versus individual determinism.

The transpersonal view of anorexia nervosa assumes that symp-

Nancy Alexander is a social worker at The Sheppard and Enoch Pratt Hospital, Towson, Maryland.

Special thanks to the following individuals for their help in preparing this paper: John Boronow, MD, The Sheppard and Enoch Pratt Hospital, Towson, Maryland 21204; Laurie Leitch, PhD, University of Maryland, Family Therapy Practice of Washington.

tom formation within family constellations represent a logical adaptation to a deviant illogical transpersonal system (Palzzoli, 1978). The symptom formation is not the end product of a series of immutable patterns or processes but a part of that system itself, functioning in an ongoing way to further both the needs, and dilemmas of that system.

In this paper, both theoretical and practical formulations are considered and integrated. Three families will be presented and discussed within their own contexts and within the theoretical constructs which so richly address this disease process both individually and systemically.

Considerable agreement exists between major theorists about a number of family characteristics although primary disagreement lies in the focus. The family systems theorists like Minuchin (1978) and Palzzoli (1978) describe the process and examine the family's communication system, its structure of leadership, its roles, and functions. Bruch (1978) and Sours (1980) tend to see the family as a collection of individuals with various personal qualities and characteristics. They describe the impact of parents on child and have identified a composite picture of both families and patients.

We will not be attempting to adjudicate between the psychoanalytic and systemic perspectives but will in the course of this presentation be applying their concepts and assessing their counterapplicability.

Bruch and Sours agree that anorexia nervosa is used to "obfuscate family conflicts in a smokescreen, and to keep parents united in concern about the child, who mediates the conflict" (Sours, p. 320). The parental relationship is empty, and it serves to entangle the potential anorexic long before she becomes symptomatic. They agree that families tend to impound affect and block expression of emotion, especially anger, and find that quiet, interminable, pseudorational arguments are the rule. Sours points out that the family "owns" the anorectic's body and sees the disorder as an effort aimed at self-ownership.

Minuchin sees the families as psychosomatic families. Such families lack normal generational boundaries, clear-cut roles, and the flexibility to adapt to the changing needs of their developing children. They expect behavior which is socially appropriate, but their children exhibit behavior which is age-appropriate (Minuchin, p. 58-60). Palzzoli addresses the problem of families coalitions—

which develop on the basis of family secrets and secret rules (Palzzoli, p. 202-215).

In an effort to examine these theorists and their views in an organized way, specific issues and problem areas will be presented in graphic form to allow the reader to compare and contrast the theories and the theorists. The characteristics have been subdivided for the readers' convenience.

In Table 1, high correlation between the four theorists can be noted. A look at inter-theorist agreement in descending order reveals that highest area of agreement was communicative, next was structure, third was interpersonal, and lowest area of agreement was in the traits section. Even in the areas where there was not consistnt agreement between the four theorists, the conclusion cannot necessarily be drawn that they do not agree, but rather that they simply have not made those observations or that they conceptualize the problem differently—systematically rather than individually. In the section where individual traits of the parents are discussed, (under Interpersonal), Minuchin and Palzzoli may not necessarily disagree with Bruch and Sours about those traits but simply think about them differently and see them as part of a systemic interaction rather than as specific personal characteristics. Within that construct, it is not that the traits do not exist, but they simply are not relevant to the theory or its application.

In some of the ratings, authors were given positive or negative ratings for specific traits, because they have addressed the issue in a similar way, not necessarily using the same exact words to describe the phenomena. For example, where Minuchin may say there is no boundary between the spousal subsystem and the child subsystem, Bruch might say that the child is overly involved in parental issues, since both would agree on the wording that the child mediates parental conflict, their intended meanings appeared to coincide, my ratings of their positions were made to reflect that similarity.

FAMILY CASE STUDIES

The theorists individually and collectively are seeking to define and describe characteristics which occur with some regularity in families which produce anorexic offspring. Each of the families described in this paper have some of the interactional characteristics

TABLE 1

CHARACTERISTICS	Bruch	Minuchin	Sours	Palazolli
Family Traits:				
perfectionistic	+	-	+	-
overconforming	+	-	+	-
emphasis on politeness	+	-	+	-
expect cheerfulness	+	-	+	-
upwardly mobile	+	-	+	-
economically secure	+	-	+	-
marriage appears stable	+	-	+	-
no violence	+	-	+	-
family small in size	+	-	+	-
mother raised children	+	-	+	-
Communication:				
conflict avoidant/detouring	+	+	+	+
avoid feelings/impound affect	+	+	+	+
discourage verbalization	+	+	+	+
crying/yelling disallowed	+	-	+	+
focus on externals	+	-	+	+
collectivity of thought	+	+	+	+
conflict underground	+	+	+	+
pseudo rational arguments	+	+	+	+
blocked expression of affect	+	+	+	+
Structure:				
enmeshed	+	+	+	+
overprotective	+	+	+	+
change resistant	+	+	+	+
parents overcontrolling	+	+	+	+
problems in leadership	-	+	-	+
problems in decision-making	-	+	-	+
confusion of needs/identity	+	-	+	-
spousal coalition weak	+	+	+	+
poor generational boundaries	+	+	+	+
problems with family of origin	+	-	+	+
Interpersonal:				
child overvalued	+	+	+	+
parents hypervigilant	+	+	+	-
overconcerned about child	+	-	+	+
parents unaffectionate with patient	+	-	+	-
parents unaffectionate with each other	+	-	+	+
marriage unsatisfying	+	+	+	+
child infantalized	+	+	+	+
child not seen as separate	+	+	+	+
child unassertive	+	+	+	+
child mediates conflicts	+	+	+	+
child overinvolved with parents	+	+	+	+
child underinvolved with peers	+	+	+	+
development seen as disloyal	+	+	+	-
lack of privacy--sex/toileting	+	+	+	+
overconcern about food/health	+	+	+	+
fear of individuation	+	+	+	+
parents intrusive with patient	+	-	+	-
father appearance-conscious	+	-	+	+
father seductive with patient	+	-	+	-
father emotionally distant	+	-	+	+
mother negative about sex	+	-	+	+
mother depressed/anhedonic	+	-	+	-
mother weight-conscious	+	-	+	-

noted by systems theorists and some of personality traits noted by analytic theorists. Yet they have their own individual issues and characteristics which make them unique.

The X Family

The X family entered treatment after the patient, Maria, a 27-year-old woman, was admitted to the hospital. She was self-referred and carried the admission diagnosis of anorexia nervosa. Her admission weight was 79 pounds. Maria, a college graduate, had been living away from home for about nine months, had obtained a college degree, and was employed in a responsible position in a large local company. Maria was embarrassed by her illness and had not visited with her parents for several months. But she was extremely emotionally dependent on them, especially her father, and talked with him on the phone at least three times a day. She had a narrow social life, was acutely symptom focused, and clinically depressed. Her history revealed binge eating without accompanying vomit/purge cycle since age 11; when last seen by parents she weighed about two hundred pounds.

The X family is a middle-class Italian family with clearly defined goals and an upwardly mobile focus. The father is a high-ranking professional, well-respected by his colleagues. The parents are from different backgrounds and differ greatly on values, attitudes, and philosophy of life. The father dominates the mother with his self-assuredness, his uncompromising stances, his intelligence, and his humor. He is concerned with his physique and appearance, always wearing several gold necklaces, and "fancy" colorful shirts. His articulation is superb, intellectual defenses flawless, and until we developed an alliance, his resistance to family therapy was formidable.

The father has a history of depression and long-standing alcoholism, coupled with reported verbal and physical spousal abuse which have been in remission for two years. The marriage is reported to have been stormy, and there have been several short separations in the past.

Mrs. X is a gentle woman, highly anxious and self-conscious, looking somewhat older than her stated years. Her dress is matronly, and she appears fragile, frazzled, fearful of saying the wrong thing, of hurting Maria, of making mistakes, or making her husband angry. A warm and engaging woman with self-effacing humor, she has a history of generalized anxiety attacks and depression, all untreated. Constantly self-conscious during the course of treatment, she began quite suddenly to diet and lost upwards of 30 pounds. She fears she will go crazy and feels guilty that she caused Maria's problems. Mrs. X feels inadequate about most things, is forgetful under stress, and resorts to writing things down that she is going to say in conversation with people. Although she is employed and well-respected in her job, her self-esteem has not improved. She believes she should never have had children because she is "unable" to be a good mother. In reality, she has been a caring mother, and her children all love her greatly.

The X family have two sons, ages 27 and 31, who both live away from home, have received college degrees, and are working in responsible positions. They too continue to be emotionally dependent on the family. Neither had started his own family at the time of initial treatment although one son became engaged during treatment and later married.

Maria was triangled in a helping role, trying to help and protect mother, trying to stop father from drinking, trying to save the marriage. She was strongly aligned in different ways with each parent. The father and Maria enjoyed a "special" relationship fraught with secrets and special nicknames. The seductiveness experienced by the patient was clearly a problem for her, and she openly acknowledged pleasure at her father's "jealousy" toward other men involved in her life.

The mother's relationship with Maria was an intense one in which there was considerable role confusion and mutual dependency. There were extensive shared confidences and the pervasive belief that Maria could save the two of them by "getting her life together."

A change in the family's roles began during the eldest son's adolescence. As the mother had grown more anxious about coping with the children, the father had moved into the role of primary parent. Through the succeeding years, the father had maintained that role while the mother had receded from the center of family life. Secrets and secret coalitions abound from this early takeover. For example, the mother was never told details of one son's legal involvements though veiled references were bantered about in her presence.

Guilt ranked high as a family emotion as did the fear of embarrassment and the fear of abandonment. Group dynamics included excessive loyalty to the nuclear family, acceptance of mutual protectiveness and overnurturance as normative, and the collective fear of changing the status-quo.

The patient felt unable to leave her mother, because her mother needed her to protect and make decisions for her. The patient felt burdened by this, but also, it gave her a sense of purpose and importance to the family unit and ensured her role in the group. Maria felt that if she were not sick and calling the family together, the group would collapse. She saw it as her duty to rescue the family. Her tie to her father was so strong that she felt unable to develop positive relationships with age-appropriate males, and as a result, most of her relationships were more fantasy than reality.

Therapy centered on freeing family members from their enmeshment, their myths, and their old family secrets, which seemed to imprison them all, on strengthening the relationship between the husband and the wife, and decentering Maria. To do this, the social worker focused on the emotional needs of the mother and gave the father specific directions about helping his wife to feel more confident. This included retraining the father to be less critical and helping him to be a better listener. We focused with Mrs. X on her self-esteem, challenging her negative self-concept, and using her childrens' attributes as reflections of her competency. Opening up communication of negative feelings so that the underground passive or symbolic communication system would be unnecessary was done through dyadic, assigned arguments, through modeling and challenging the father, then encouraging the sons to do the same. Praise and support was given when people were open and clear about their feelings. The inclusion of both male siblings encouraged decentralization of the patient and discouraged triangulation with the parents. They were able to validate Maria's views of the problems and to normalize some of her perceptions. Also, because of their willingness to confront father, they helped their mother and Maria increase their skills in dealing with their father.

One intervention allowed the family to test out its new-found competence at several family dinners in which conflictual topics were assigned; they found that they could disagree angrily without disaster. The realization that they could safely disagree was reframed as an autonomy issue, such that the children felt freer to leave home emotionally without fear of family dissolution.

The issue of individual rather than collective responsibility was most dramatically crystalized in a "mock funeral" which followed Maria's discussion of her suicidal feelings and ended with the firm acknowledgement that Maria's life was her own.

The Y Family

The Y family entered treatment shortly after Jeffrey, 21, the oldest son in a sib system of four, entered the hospital in an acute psychotic episode. The family was a middle-class, Jewish, single-parent family headed by the father. The Mother had died two years prior as a result of a brain aneurism. The anoretic in the family, Shelly, age 19, the second oldest child, had been hospitalized three times previously in medium-length facilities for anorexia. She was not following through with her aftercare plans. During the course of her brother's hospitalization, she was seen in family therapy, and individually, for the purpose of developing a referral for long-term individual psychotherapy. The other sibs in the family were Mark, age 17, who was a reported alcoholic and was described as "out of control," and Amy, 16, who was described as problem-free. She attended Catholic Prep School, worked at a restaurant, and volunteered as a paramedic with a local fire department.

The father, Mr. Y, was work-worn, overwhelmed, highly anxious, and occasionally presented thought-disorder and paranoia. His decision-making style was one of passive leadership: He would let the kids "fight it out" and decide by default or would make arbitrary decisions based on concrete details like money or the weather. He was employed in a local company as a researcher and had had to abandon his plans to be a doctor due to his mother's long-term illness. His presenting style was of passive-dependency, and long-suffering martyrdom.

Mrs. Y, deceased, lived most of her adult life as an invalid. She had been diagnosed with multiple sclerosis shortly after Jeffrey's birth, but there were some signs of her illness prior to the marriage. Her personality and style of leadership, described by the family and interwoven with specific features of the illness itself, was one of intense emotional overinvolvement with the children, marked by rage reactions when her needs or decisions were not responded to immediately. Throughout her life, her condition deteriorated drastically, and Shelly became her primary caretaker from age 11. She was responsible for helping mother bathe, fixing her hair, and was involved in a whole range of self-care activities. Father consistently deferred to his wife such that the whole household revolved around the sickbed and an unstable, labile, deeply despondent woman, whose life-death wishes were erratic.

Mrs. Y's death was shocking and traumatic to the family. No grieving took place, and the family members never discussed her death or the impact it had on their lives. They never discussed her illness in anything other than practical terms, like dates, doctors' names, and procedures performed such that affect around her illness and her death was significantly blocked. No consensual validation or sharing of conflictual feelings had ever taken place, and family members were becoming strangers to each other: Their conversation was superficial, their real feelings were hidden, their movements seemed stiff and constrained. Even the content of their fights was avoidant, as they focused on concrete externals with raging emotions.

Mr. Y depended heavily on Shelly for functional tasks. She was in most ways the new female head of household. She cooked, shopped, cleaned, held the credit cards, and managed everyone's schedules. Shelly's position was not recognized by her siblings, who fought with her about being in charge and mocked her about her anorexia. The sibling system developed a street pack quality, in which there was considerable infighting and battling for power, and yet a high level of loyalty was presented to the outside world. Their concern for each other played itself out by "tattling" on one another and by pressuring father to take various "punishing" positions.

The family suffered from lack of leadership and unresolved emotional issues around mother's long-standing illness and traumatic death. There was significant role confusion and role distortion, and consensus around the most basic issues was impossible. Family members felt demoralized about their sick members and about family functioning in general. All children except Jeffrey had found "other families" with whom they spent time and shared idealistic "good family" fantasies. The family's collective transference was a maternal one, and there was a strong pull from the group to have the therapist take over the care and management of the family. The efforts and maneuvers in this regard were endless and became the focal point of many of the sessions.

Shelly had identified with her sick and dying mother, who had lost great amounts of weight and before her death had become emaciated. The closeness and the care-taking role appeared to have led to identity confusion for Shelly and to profound body image problems. She felt burdened now with the family and more specifically with her father's dependency needs. She was angry and fearful about her siblings' problems and about her father's growing inadequacies and demands on her. She fended off her fears about the sexuality implicit between them by extreme weight loss, noncompliance with treatment, and continuous hostile arguments with him about decisions he made or failed to make.

Therapy with the family addressed the issue of leadership and decision-making. Efforts were made to develop a set of "house rules" and to help father to enforce them. The children were asked to take turns helping father with enforcement as a way of helping father to take charge and and of helping Shelly to disengage. The father was encouraged to make independent decisions without relying on the sibling group for input.

In working with the Y's, it became clear that the family was tightly organized around illness, which kept the father and children tied to each other. A more competency-based focus was needed. Interventions began with several reframes in an effort to reorganize the family toward relationships outside the household. The freeing reframe for father, who was most resistant, was a sacrificial one which echoed his personal style and urged him to "go out with other adults" for the sake of the children.

Because of its centrality as an issue, a memorial service for the mother was developed which took place in the office. The service included the use of photographs and a structured affective approach which involved writing positive and negative memories about mother in response to specifically designed questions. This helped family members to reconstruct their history together and to surface issues and conflicts vis-à-vis mother. The ceremony was a sharing moment for the family, involving real exchanges of feeling; and it allowed for clarification, validation and some resolution.

Next, Shelly was encouraged to disengage, to stay in the dormitory at college rather than to drive home each day, and encouraged to develop a social life. In this regard, the sisters were instructed to go out socially together which reinforced their alliance with each other and allowed Amy to model for Shelly.

Helping the family to deal with Mark was more difficult. He was actively rebellious, and direct work on improving the parent-child relationship was complicated by father's unyielding negative attitude toward Mark as well as by Mark's concrete thinking and oppositional behavior. Eventually, arrangements were made for him to live with his grandmother, and later, he moved into on-campus housing.

Amy, who had remained essentially uninvolved in many of the family conflicts, was able to gain early admission to college and moved into on-campus housing just prior to the end of the family therapy.

Because of the nature of the problems and the father's inadequacies, an insight-oriented approach was not used. Interventions were structural, strategic, and practical in nature although the therapeutic bond between the therapist and the children was central to the work and seemed at times to provide them with the motivation for attending the sessions.

The Z Family

The Z family came into treatment shortly after Rebecca, age 27, was admitted for her first hospitalization, diagnosed with anorexia nervosa and weighing 68 pounds. She was the fourth of seven siblings born to a wealthy upper-class Jewish family. Her natural father to whom she had been especially close had died when she was seven. His death had not been discussed, grieved, nor had any of the children been allowed to attend the funeral. The mother thought it best not to discuss unpleasantness and had remarried shortly after his death to a man bearing the same name as her dead husband.

Mrs. Z is seen by her children as all powerful and controlling. She had had a troubled childhood relationship with her own mother, which had not been resolved and which she was reluctant to discuss in depth. Mrs. Z had been abusive to her children, hitting them repeatedly, pushing them into objects or down the stairs. When younger, the children were fearful of her and sought her approval. Because of their great demands as well as the mother's fears and conflicts over the children, a series of housekeepers were employed to care for them. She demanded obedience and compliance from the children about trivial issues, and she was concerned about social status and social adequacy. She had developed a forbidding facade wherein she appeared strong and autocratic but which served to cover her deep insecurities and feelings of inadequacy.

Mrs. Z's behavior with the hospital staff was demanding and short sighted, and although care was taken to provide her with great amounts of information about the treatment and the illness, she failed to absorb this information and insisted that the solutions to Rebecca's problems were simple ones, i.e., get her to eat ice cream. She angrily protested more complex solutions or explanations and returned perseveratively to her original perspective. Throughout the hospitalization, the mother complained about treatment programming and threatened repeatedly to take her daughter out of the hospital; during the course of treatment, the mother lost 20 pounds.

Mr. Z was a wealthy, well-intentioned man, who was extremely dependent on his wife and somatically preoccupied to the point of hypochondriasis. His feelings of anxiety and inadequacy were palpable. Quickly moved to tears, he was fearful about his relationship with the children in the family. Mrs. Z defended him furiously and was enraged about the children's reactions to him. In their early years together, he was seen by the children as another child, whose behavior was described as manipulative, and he resorted to techniques, such as threats and bribery, in order to gain control over the sibling group. True parent-child relationships never developed; the parents felt that the children were responsible for this.

Historically, Rebecca was "the runt of the litter," rejected by mother from birth for reasons of appearance. She was a quiet child, greatly overpowered by her six noisy, competent, outgoing siblings. She felt she had never had a relationship with her mother although she longed for one. She spent her life "slipping through the cracks" and had developed a "last-in-line" attitude, even in regard to food. She rarely asked for seconds and established a self-deprivation cycle early in life. She formed strong attachments to her older, more accomplished siblings, who in turn looked out for her and allowed her to tag along with them. In adult life, those relationships were central to her although she struggled with issues of closeness and isolation.

The sibling group itself was complex and impressive. One of the female siblings had long since broken off relations with the family except for occasional contact with one brother. She was a source of considerable pain to the family, and much time was spent discussing her loss. The siblings, ranging from mid 20's to late 30's, were bright, accomplished, well-educated, and competent. They were established in careers, two in the helping professions, and several had married. They were uniquely able to participate in the family therapy sessions to structure and use the time effectively and to deal with current problematic issues and issues.

The earliest therapeutic intervention focused on shifting group attention from the patient's symptoms to looking at the family as a group. The clarification of hierarchy and roles led to an understanding of the family's processes and to identifying individual identities in this large family system. It became clear that there was a strong, informal system in which many of the parental roles had been subdivided among the children. The mother's apparent autocracy was maintained as a myth while the emotional and nurturant roles had been taken over by several of the older girls in the family. This was largely unrecognized, and the girls in the family felt undersupported by mother, who in turn felt unappreciated by them and wished to receive care and nurturance from them the way the younger children did. Once the family members felt free to discuss these issues, they became involved in active problem solving and moved to realign and to revise roles in more age-appropriate and growth-producing ways. They set limits on Rebecca's expectations and redefined the parental role in more realistic ways. The family was reframed as adaptive, and members were encouraged to take pride in their growth rather than resist it.

Historic issues, such as father's death, the child abuse, and the step-father's role in the family were strongly felt in their unresolved states, and efforts were made to provide a forum for their discussion and resolution. The therapist role here was that of moderator and commentator. Common problems were validated as they arose, and communication skills were taught with an emphasis on active listening and assertiveness in communication.

From Rebecca's point of view, the sessions were an opportunity to get some of the attention she had never had. Parents and siblings traveled thousands of miles from five different states monthly for three-hour marathon sessions. She was the center. Initially, she regressed, behaving in a passive, tearful manner as mother and step-father asked her personal questions about her food intake and bodily functioning. The dual issues of privacy and choice were highlighted for her, and she was encouraged to keep her bodily issues secret and to decide what information she wanted to share with her parents and her siblings. Through this process, she was able to be assertive in warding off unwanted intrusion and in developing an increasing sense of self-control. Her siblings were most useful in this process, serving as role models and as a support to encourage her new-found competence.

With encouragement, the mother began to express some of her

hidden feelings. She emerged in a more vulnerable and real way with the result that the children were now able to be both affectionte and assertive with her.

DISCUSSION

Though they vary greatly in nature, personality, and degree of internal dysfunction, each of these families have some similar characteristics in common. However, they vary greatly with some of the standard biodemographic data generally thought to be true of families with anorexic offspring. Families are thought to be typically upwardly mobile and economically secure. Although this was true of two families, the Y family would not fit that description; although the father valued success and education, members were not necessarily encouraged to pursue an education, and finances was a constant worry for them. It is generally thought that there are a few broken homes in these families, yet the X family had been through a number of separations, and both the Y and Z families had had parental deaths with Mrs. Z having remarried. Two of the marriages described could not be seen as conventional or stable, X because of overt marital problems, alcoholism, and spousal abuse, Y because of Mrs. Y's debilitating illness and subsequent dysfunction, wherein her mental stability was in serious question, and the spousal relationship was imbalanced. The Z marriage while appearing to be internally functional was clearly problematic within the family context.

Families of anorectic offspring have a solid reputation for lack of overt arguments and lack of violence, and yet each of the families reported here have histories of violence. X had spousal abuse. Y had documented child abuse from the mother as well as occasional violence between the siblings. The Z family also had a history of child abuse from mother and reported incidents of violence between the children beyond what might be considered normal limits.

All our families were larger than is considered normative for these families (2.8 children), and all families contained male offspring although the literature indicates that there is paucity of sons in families which produce anorectic offspring. Despite the fact that mothers of anorectic children are known to take great pride in their child-raising abilities and children are rarely raised by surrogates, the Z children had a series of maids and housekeepers who cared for them, and because of their mother's illness, the Y children were cared for in part by their grandmothers. Mrs. X, who did raise her own children, did not take pride in her accomplishment and in fact felt a failure because of it.

One might conclude from this that these families are perhaps atypical, and their additional life stresses, complications, and variance with the established normative patterns may in some way account for the seriousness of the patient's disorders and for some of the difficulties encountered in treating these families.

FAMILY CHARACTERISTIC CHART

The list of characteristics represents qualities which have been identified by four major theorists as characteristics of families with anorexic offspring. It allows the reader to see how/when/where those qualities apply to the three families described. No single family uniformly met "the stereotype," though as a group, they scored high and met most of the qualities listed. The scoring for each family on each charactristic listed is subjective and is meant to reflect an overall impression of the family based on that characteristic at the beginning of treatment. Some of the scores would be altered because of changes made during treatment although effectiveness of treatment is not being evaluated in this paper. Qualities which would have affected symptom formation are the focus, and traits are scored as they were at time of assessment. Some of the scoring is additionally limited, as in the case of Mrs. Y, because it is based on second-hand information. In instances where there is great variation on a given trait between individuals in a family, the parents and patient are scored for that characteristic. (See Table 2.)

Families were rated on 51 possible traits (variables) in an effort to see how these families compared with the standard for families with anorectic offspring.

The highest consensus among the families was in the communications section in which all three families combined received 85 percent positive scores indicating high incidence of defined communication problems in the families.

In the section on family structure, there were also significant positive ratings. In this section out of the possible traits listed, the families as a group scored 76.7 percent positive.

In the interpersonal section, there was a high degree of variance.

TABLE 2

CHARACTERISTICS	X	Y	Z
Family Traits:			
perfectionistic	+	-	-
overconforming	+	+	+
emphasis on politeness	+	-	+
expect cheerfulness	-	-	+
upwardly mobile	+	-	+
economically secure	+	-	+
marriage appears stable	-	-	+
no violence	-	-	-
family small in size	-	-	-
mother raised children	+	-	-
Communication:			
conflict avoidant/detouring	+	+	+
avoid feelings/impound affect	+	+	+
discourage verbalization	+	+	+
crying/yelling disallowed	+	-	+
focus on externals	-	+	+
collectivity of thought	-	+	+
conflict underground	+	+	+
pseudo rational arguments	+	-	+
blocked expression of affect	+	+	+
Structure:			
enmeshed	+	+	+
overprotective	+	-	-
change resistant	+	+	+
parents overcontrolling	+	-	+
problems in leadership	-	+	+
problems in decision-making	+	+	+
confusion of needs/identity	+	+	-
spousal coalition weak	+	N/A	-
poor generational boundaries	+	+	-
problems with family of origin	+	+	+
Interpersonal:			
child overvalued	+	+	-
parents hypervigilant	+	-	-
overconcerned about child	+	-	-
parents unaffectionate with patient	-	+	+
parents unaffectionate with each other	+	N/A	-
marriage unsatisfying	+	N/A	-
child infantalized	+	-	+
child not seen as separate	+	+	+
child unassertive	+	+	+
child mediates conflicts	+	+	-
child overinvolved with parents	+	+	-
child underinvolved with peers	+	+	+
development seen as disloyal	+	+	+
lack of privacy--sex/toileting	-	+	
overconcern about food/health	-	+	+
fear of individuation	+	+	+
parents intrusive with patient	+	+	+
father appearance-conscious	+	-	+
father seductive with patient	+	-	+
father emotionally distant	-	+	-
mother negative about sex	+	N/A	+
mother depressed/anhedonic	+	+	-
mother weight-conscious	+	+	+

We found the 66 percent were rated positive with a high degree of variance between the families.

The family traits section showed the least amount of conformity with the standard for families with patients in this diagnostic group with a positive rating of only 48 percent.

Looking at the data from an individual family perspective, one finds that out of 51 possible traits, the X family most closely met the "stereotype" with 11 negative ratings and 40 positive ratings. The Z family had 18 negative ratings leaving 33 positive ratings, and the Y family had 19 negative ratings, four N/A, and 28 positive ratings. (See Figure 1.)

The positive (presence of a characteristic) or negative (absence of a characteristic) ratings do not specifically correlate with nor are they meant to imply health or illness in the family system. When viewed from a functional perspective, the family most closely associated with the standard is the X family, which showed a high degree of strength and improvement during the treatment process. Conversely, the family who proved to be furthest from the standard developed here was the Y family, and that family showed the highest degree of disorganization throughout the treatment process.

In reflecting on these ratings, other issues and factors, such as parental illness and death, are relevant but have not been listed. These two factors existed in two of the families presented and may have contributed to the development of anorexia more than listed characteristics. In such instances, one might consider that anorexia might develop from an entirely different constellation of factors and issues.

Regarding conclusions about this data, it is noted that the highest areas of consistency, not only among the family groups but also among the theorists, was in the area of communication in which four theorists agreed with each other about the various communication traits 28 to two. It must be emphasized that disagreement between theorists may simply mean that no position was taken on that trait by that theorist.

It is interesting that there is low agreement in the family traits section in which out of a possible 40, the theorists are split 20/20 paralleling the low findings in that section for the family group.

In this regard, one might speculate that the higher level of theoretical agreement there is about a specific point or subset, the higher likelihood there is that those factors will prove to be clinically valid.

In summation although different theorists approached the prob-

FIGURE I

FAMILY CHARACTERISTICS COMPARISON CHART

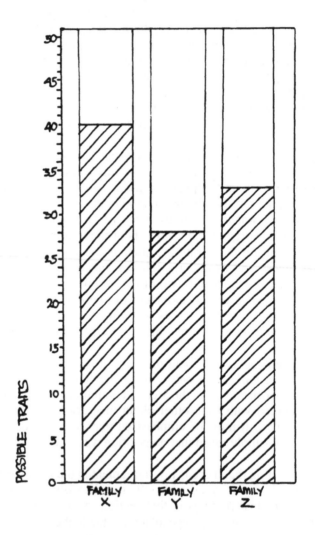

lem from different viewpoints, there was still a high degree of agreement about the families which produce anorexic offspring. In spite of the fact that different words were often used to described the traits or exchange processes, it was clear the systems theorists and analysts alike were viewing and trying to describe essentially the same collection of intrafamilial phenomena.

In detailing these three families, an effort was made to apply theory about family structure, process, and characteristics to clinical practice. Families were alike structurally, but the greatest similarity occurred in the area of communication. Because of the small sample under discussion, no sweeping conclusions can be made, but further attention should be directed to communications theory and to creative thought about the origins of such problems and about possible applications for treatment in this family diagnostic group.

REFERENCES

Bruch, H., M.D. (1978). *The Golden Cage: The Enigma of Anorexia Nervosa.* Cambridge: Harvard University.

Minuchin, S., Rosman, B., and Baker, L. (1978) *Psychosomatic Families: Anorexia Nervosa in Context.* Cambridge: Harvard University.

Palzzoli, M.S. (1978). *Self Starvation.* New York: J. Aronson.

Sours, J.A., M.D. (1980). *Starving to Death in a Sea of Objects: The Anorexia Nervosa Syndrome,* New York: Jason Aronson.

OTHER SUGGESTED READINGS

Crisp, A. H. (1979). Early Recognition and Prevention of Anorexia Nervosa. *Developmental Medicine and Child Neurology, 21,* 393-395.

Goetz, P. L., M.D., Succop, R. A., A.C.S.W., Reinhart, J. B., M.D. and Miller, A., M.D. (1977. Anorexia Nervosa in Children: A Follow-up Study. *American Journal of Orthopsychiatry, 47*(4), 597-603.

Halmijk, A., M.D., Struss, A., M.D. and Goldberg, S. C., M.D. (1978). Brief Communication: An Investigation of Weights in the Parents of Anorexia Nervosa Patients. *The Journal of Nervous and Mental Disease,* 166(5) 358-361.

Mintz, I. L., M.D. (1980), Anorexia Nervosa: The Clinical Syndrome and Its Dynamic Implications. *Journal of The Medical Society of N.J.,* 77(5) 341-344.

Norris, D. L. (1979). Clinical Diagnostic Criteria for Primary Anorexia Nervosa: An Analysis of 54 Consecutive Admissions. *South African Medical Journal, 56,* 987-993.

Rampling, D. (1980). Single Case Study: Abnormal Mothering in the Genesis of Anorexia Nervosa. *The Journal of Nervous and Mental Disease, 168*(8), 501-5021.

Rickaeby, G. A. (1979). Psychosocial Dynamics in Anorexia Nervosa. *The Medical Journal of Australia, 1,* 587-589.

Wilson, C. P., M.D. (1980). The Family Psychological Profile of Anorexia Nervosa Patients. *Journal of The Medical Society of N.J.,* 77(5), 333-339.

Yager, J., M.D. (1982). Family Issues in The Pathogenesis of Anorexia Nervosa. *Psychosomatic Medicine, 44*(1), 43-60.

When Doing Is Not Enough:
The Relationship Between Activity and Effectiveness in Anorexia Nervosa

M. A. McColl, BSc, MHSc
J. Friedland, BA, MA, OT(C)
A. Kerr, BSc (OT)

ABSTRACT. The prevalence of anorexia nervosa is increasing throughout the world, both clinically and sub-clinically (Crisp, 1976; Jones, 1980). Occupational therapists are often involved in the treatment of these women, especially with regard to development of the sense of effectiveness. Application of fundamental occupational therapy principles suggests that the prescription of activity should help anorexics to develop individual competencies, which would subsequently generalize into a sense of effectiveness over time (Fidler, 1981). However, experience with anorexics in an inpatient treatment unit has challenged this basic assumption. The paper is an attempt to understand and explain the relationships among three factors: anorexia, the sense of ineffectiveness, and the use and meaning of activity. Attempts are made to explain the development of the sense of effectiveness in healthy people, and discussion targets the areas where this process may break down in the anorexic. A detailed discussion of activity and past research on activity demonstrates the state of knowledge on this topic within the field of occupational therapy, and pinpoints the need for further research to more appropriately utilize activity in the remediation of the sense of ineffectiveness, particularly with anorexics.

Anorexia nervosa is an eating disorder characterized by an intense fear of becoming fat, disturbance of body image, significant weight loss, amenorrhea in women and refusal to maintain normal body weight (DSM III, 1980, p. 67). The most well known studies by Crisp (1976) and Jones (1980) document the increasing preva-

M. A. McColl and J. Friedland are Assistant Professors in the Department of Rehabilitation Medicine, University of Toronto. A. Kerr is a lecturer in the Department of Psychiatry, University of Toronto. He is also Senior Occupational Therapist at Toronto General Hospital.

137

lence of the disorder from 1% to 3% in young women. Anorexic
"behaviour", or subclinical forms of anorexia nervosa, in the general population are cited to be on a similar increase at a prevalence
of 10 to 14% (Garfinkel and Garner, 1982). Despite the changing
statistics for prevalence, the sex distribution of the disorder has remained constant at 90 to 95% female (Bemis, 1980).

With the increasing number of cases coming to the attention of
general and psychiatric facilities, the demand for specialized treatment of this sometimes fatal disorder cannot be ignored. There is
agreement that the origins of anorexia are multi-determined; that is,
the disorder is a consequence of biological, psychological and social
factors. As a result, interventions have developed at individual,
family and cultural levels. In the case of the treatment team, the efforts are multidisciplinary, often requiring the expertise of psychiatrists, psychologists, social workers, nurses, nutritionists and occupational therapists (Garfinkel and Garner, 1982).

Still fundamental to the understanding of the disorder, is one of
the psychological constructs put forth by Bruch (1973). She identified the "pervasive sense of ineffectiveness" and subsequent lack
of personal identity as a core predisposition to the illness. Anorexic
patients "experience themselves as not being in control of their
behaviour, needs and impulses, as not owning their own bodies, as
not having a sense of gravity within themselves. Instead they feel
under the influence and direction of external forces. They act as if
their own body and behaviour were the product of other people's influences and actions" (Bruch, 1973, p. 55). Bruch's central theme
is that the search for self-control and autonomy is maladaptively
pursued through control over one's body, in particular, one's
weight.

Paradoxically, as the anorexic succeeds in her pursuit of thinness,
she loses control over other aspects of her life. She loses concentration and becomes intensely preoccupied with thoughts of food; she
becomes fearful of losing control of her emotions; she is irritable,
and experiences lowered self-esteem and increased social isolation.
Other aggravating symptoms of starvation may drive her to seek
help and hospitalization, e.g. faintness, muscle cramps or gastrointestinal problems.

Hospitalization is considered necessary in order to restore normal
eating behaviours, to promote psychological development, and to
break the vicious diet cycle. Strategies at this phase of the treatment
in many centres are behavioural: privileges are contingent on weight

gain, there is gradual desensitization to "phobic" foods, weights, and clothing sizes, and behaviour is shaped away from food-related preoccupations.

At Toronto General Hospital, an Inpatient Eating Disorder Unit was formed in 1982. Four beds out of twenty were put aside on a general psychiatric floor for the care of the eating disordered patient. A well-defined behavioural program was designed by a multidisciplinary team. The program consists of a pre-admission assessment, an observation period of one to two weeks, a treatment phase of several months in which all privileges are contingent on weight gain, and a final period of weight stabilization, when the transfer into the community of newly acquired eating behaviours and attitudes toward food is ensured.

The role of occupational therapy is to design an individualized program for each patient. Privileges which are believed to have reinforcing properties are made contingent on weight gain. For instance, weight gain of one kilogram would be rewarded by an additional bedrest activity and telephone privileges. The assumption is that activities are enjoyable and desirable and that to have the activities is better than not having activities. A second assumption is that the successful completion of activities will ameliorate the impaired sense of effectiveness. Control over bodily functions will be exerted instead over objects.

In the early stages of treatment, the assumptions made about activities seem to bear out. Patients respond to the contingencies and work hard for their privileges. In the later stage of treatment, when activities are unlimited, observations made by occupational therapists call into question the function of activities for these women. Despite prolific and excellent performance on activities, e.g. knitting, calligraphy and bead work, these women do not report feelings of satisfaction or effectiveness. Instead, they regard the successful completion of activities as somewhat irrelevant, and comments that would be regarded as socially reinforcing (e.g., "That's wonderful", "You've done a great job") are received with mistrust (e.g., "What do you mean?", "Why do you say that?"). These observations are made in stark contrast to the kind of experiences other patients seem to have upon the successful completion of activities. For other patient groups, the successful completion of activities represents to both the staff and patients themselves, a movement towards health and the resolution of their illness. Competencies and skills reflect well-being, and this is borne out in self reports by patients.

These observations have led the authors to question some of our assumptions about activities. Do activities have intrinsic properties that will be revealed as one does the activity? Is there an interface between the activity and the experience of doing an activity? Is the anorexic population unique in its response to activities?

ANOREXIA AND THE SENSE OF INEFFECTIVENESS

It has been suggested by Bruch (1973) that anorexics experience a pervasive sense of ineffectiveness. This feeling of ineffectiveness may be first noted in descriptions of anorexics as children. They are generally described as compliant children, not disruptive nor rebellious, not particularly imaginative nor creative, not risk-taking nor adventurous (Bruch, 1979). They are seen as model children, never giving their parents or teachers a moment's concern. It is as though they fear for their survival should they choose to exert their own will and be the origins of their own behaviour.

The idea that one is the origin of one's behaviour has been explored and developed by DeCharms (1968) through the concept of personal causation. He defines personal causation as "the desire to be master of one's fate" (p. 270), and he goes on to further describe it as,

> an overarching or guiding principle upon which specific motives are built. The environment sets different problems (obtaining food, achieving success, gaining friendship, etc.) that may help to define specific motives for individual behaviour patterns. The dimension that underlies all of these is the attempt to overcome the problem through personal causation (p. 270). Personal causation is not a specific motive, because it involves no specific goal, but can apply to the means of attaining any objective goal. (p. 271).

DeCharms (1968) emphasizes the important subjective quality of the concept of personal causation. He coins the terms "Origin" and "Pawn" to describe people in terms of their perception of the locus of causation of events in their environment. In the following definitions he makes a distinction between the feeling state of the Origin and the feeling state of the Pawn. An Origin is defined as someone with "a strong feeling of personal causation, a feeling that the locus for causation of effects in his environment lies within himself"

(p. 274). "A Pawn", he states, "has a feeling that causal forces beyond his control, or personal forces residing in others, or in the physical environment, determine his behaviour, and this constitutes a strong feeling of powerlessness or ineffectiveness" (p. 274). This important concept has been brought into the occupational therapy literature in a classic paper by Burke (1977). The sense of ineffectiveness found in the Pawn appears to be very similar to that expressed by Bruch (1973) in describing the anorexic.

Given the description of the typical anorexic's childhood put forward earlier (Bruch, 1973), it is assumed that the sense of effectiveness is not present at an early stage in her development. Piaget (1952) implies that to feel effective, or to feel that one can make an impact upon one's world, requires an opportunity to do so. White (1971) further suggests that a valuing or respect by others for the actions so taken is required for development of the sense of effectiveness. The environment should therefore provide opportunities for activity, and reinforcement that activity has had an impact (whether positive or negative). The environment should be pliable in the sense that it can respond to the actions of the individual. It should allow for exploratory behaviour where there are no life-threatening risks or consequences.

This clearly does not describe the early environment typical of anorexic women. Instead, Bruch (1985) describes that environment as "seemingly well-functioning homes [where parents] raise children who mistrust their ability to face the future and shy away from adult living. On one level, child care appears to be excellent, everything is provided for, materially, psychologically, and culturally. However, little attention is paid to the child's expression of needs, wants, and feelings" (p.10). Thus, while learning or skill development occurs in these young girls, the environment is not sufficiently plastic to allow the perception of having had an impact or of having made a difference. This idea helps to explain the failure in development of the sense of effectiveness in the anorexic.

Anorexics are frequently described as being high achievers, people with considerable skill and ability, above average in scholastic achievement. Objectively, they may indeed be "competent", i.e. "sufficient or adequate to meet the demands of a situation or task" (White, 1971, p. 273). To be of value to an individual, however, this objective capacity for success must be accompanied by a subjetive belief in that capacity. It is the belief in competence which is lacking in the anorexic.

White (1959) has dealt with this link between competence and effectiveness in his landmark paper, entitled, "Motivation Reconsidered". Although the major focus of that work was to re-define and extend the understanding of motivation, he also introduced the concept of competence. Competence, he suggested, resulted from what he labelled as "effectance motivation". Effectance motivation was described as one's striving for the *feeling* of effectiveness and not just for the results of one's efforts. Effectance motivation was thought to take an undifferentiated form in early childhood, (i.e., exploratory behaviour) similar to that described by Piaget (1952) in his many observations of his infants' joy at having exerted an influence on their environment. The same process of effectance motivation is later distinguished as various specific motives, including those of mastery and achievement (White, 1959).

Bandura (1977) examines the concept of effectiveness from a slightly different perspective, under what he calls efficacy expectation. Efficacy expectation is defined as "the conviction that one can successfully execute the behaviour required to produce the outcomes" (p. 193). This expectation is reinforced by an experience arising from successful performance. Bandura points out that "expectation alone will not produce desired performance if the component capabilities are lacking" (p. 194). This, however, is not the problem experienced by anorexics, who seem to possess the component capabilities, but have no experience of effectiveness or expectation of success.

It would appear then that there is a cyclical aspect involved in the workings of these concepts of competence and effectiveness. The motivation for effectance, as White describes it, sets the stage for learning and developing competencies. Competencies, so developed, reinforce the expectation of effectiveness, and thereby, the expectation of success (Bandura, 1977). The efficacy expectation then allows effectance motivation to stimulate further initiatives, leading to a broader range of competencies.

White (1971) addressed the issue of interdependence of the concepts when he discussed "the human being as a system . . . in itself a source of influence as well as shaped by outside influences" (p. 272). What he is describing here is the idea of the human being as a open system, influenced by feedback processes both internal and external to the organism. This idea has been well-developed in the occupational therapy literature dealing with General Systems Theory (Kielhofner, 1978).

There has been a tendency to group together the concepts of competence and the sense of effectiveness in the occupational therapy literature. Fidler (1981) has quite rightly pointed out the interrelatedness of the concepts of competency, mastery, achievement, self-esteem, self value and worth. However, despite their similarities, there are important differences between these concepts, and unfortunately, consistent terminology has not been maintained, and the complex inter-relationships between them has not been fully unravelled.

Fidler (1981) states that the innate drive toward mastery is "essential to survival and that it is critical for defining and verifying one's competence, ability to overcome, to manage, to perform, and therefore to be able to make an impact on one's world" (p. 569). With such a statement, attention is focussed on competence as a reinforcer of the sense of effectiveness. Fidler (1981) further states that, the sense of effectiveness or inner assurance comes from an accumulation of objective experiences of competence, and the "larger the aggregate of masteries, the more solid and all-pervasive, the sense of competence" (p. 569).

The development or re-establishment of competence is a primary goal in occupational therapy for a number of different patient groups. In theory, "doing" will in itself provide a patient with a sense of having an impact on his world, and "doing more" will result in an all-pervasive sense of competence (Fidler, 1978). However, for some populations, for example, anorexics, unless the reinforcing link exists between competence and perceived effectiveness, such an approach will serve only to increase the objective reality of competence, without its equally important subjective component of *belief* in competence, or the sense of effectiveness.

WHEN DOING IS NOT ENOUGH

In Fidler's 1981 article, entitled, "From crafts to competence", she describes 6 assumptions on which the use of purposeful activity by occupational therapists is based.

1. First, activities are assumed to be weighted based on their social value. Therefore some tasks have a greater potential to promote adaptation than others, due to the extent to which they are recognized socially.

2. Second, an individual's abilities make some tasks more successful and gratifying than others. These tasks are therefore more successful in promoting competence.
3. Activities have certain real and symbolic meanings.
4. Activities have distinguishable psychomotor components, which can be isolated and identified.
5. The degree to which an activity is successfully matched with a patient's needs determines the success of that activity for remediation.
6. Finally, the sense of mastery in an activity is related to the end product or result.

Clinical observations with anorexia challenge assumptions 2 and 6. Despite high levels of performance and "better than average" end products, these competencies do not have the hypothesized cumulative effect, leading to a feeling of effectiveness. This fact makes assumptions 1, 3 and 5 particularly interesting, and worthy of deeper understanding. What are the social meanings that we attach to activity? What are the symbolic or underlying meanings of activity to various clients? And how can we better understand what activities offer, in an effort to better match them with patients needs?

USE OF ACTIVITY IN OCCUPATIONAL THERAPY

Activities have been used by occupational therapists for a variety of therapeutic purposes throughout the history of the profession. Bissell and Mailloux (1981) call activities, or more specificially, crafts, "a central concept in occupational therapy since the founding of the profession" (p. 369). Activities are defined in a recent position paper by AOTA as "tasks or experiences in which the person actively participates" (Hinojosa, Sabari and Rosenfeld, 1983, p. 805). Crafts are further defined as "tangible objects produced from resource materials, such as clay, yarn, leather or wood" (Bissell and Mailloux, 1981, p. 371). Crafts are differentiated from many other occupational therapy activities by the fact that they result in a tangible end product, which provides empirical evidence of success or failure.

The idea of activity or occupation is mentioned in almost every definition or statement about occupational therapy, from the classic Reilly quote:

Man, through the use of his hands, as they are energized by the mind and will, can influence the state of his own health. (Reilly, 1962, p.2)

to the official AOTA definition of occupational therapy:

The art and science of directing man's participation in selected activity . . . (Engelhardt, 1977, p. 667)

Occupational therapy, on this continent, had its organized beginnings in the very early 20th century. The focus on activity at that time was an extension of the moral treatment philosophy prevalent during the century before. At its origin, crafts and diversional activity were the main focus of occupational therapy. There have been a number of articles in the recent literature, tracing the role of activity through the early development of occupational therapy and emphasizing the importance of occupation as a unifying concept (Kielhofner and Burke, 1977; Gillette and Kielhofner, 1979; Bissell and Mailloux, 1981; Shannon, 1977). Throughout our history, the significance of the use of crafts as therapeutic activity has varied, reaching a low in recent years, concurrent with the trend towards mechanization and technologization of health care. A U.S. survey, by Bissell and Mailloux in 1981, showed that 28% of therapists polled did not use crafts at all in their practice, and that a further 37% used crafts less than 20% of the time. The reasons stated for non-use were difficulty in justifying craft use to patients and other professionals, and lack of precision in documenting change based on craft activities. These objections underline the need for further research to assist in understanding the therapeutic use of crafts in occupational therapy. Shannon (1977) states that the present devaluation of crafts as therapeutic activities is evidence of the "derailment of occupational therapy". He uses the term derailment to refer to a departure from basic principles and values, and he encourages occupational therapists towards a re-commitment to fundamental ideals.

Activity analysis is the basic tool used by occupational therapists to match patient needs with the need-fulfilling capacities of activity. Kremer, Nelson and Duncombe (1984), however, pose the question whether therapists can legitimately assume that patients have the same reactions to activity as those on which activity analysis is based (i.e., those of the therapist). Given the centrality of the use of activity and activity analysis to occupational therapy, the literature on this topic is surprisingly sparse, and largely intuitive in nature. The following is a review of the occupational therapy literature on activity and activity analysis, with emphasis on the approach to activity and attempts to understand its meaning.

The early literature on activity analysis employed a psychodynamic approach. Fidler's classic 1948 article outlined the various psychological constructs that could be examined and attributed to activity. Her approach revolved primarily around the varying capacity of activities to provide expression, gratification and sublimation of repressed drives or emotions.

Taber, Baron and Blackwell (1953) used a similar method in analyzing 29 activities. Activities were classifed according to their ability to provide expression for hostility, aggression or narcissism, to expiate guilt or to soothe, stimulate or challenge patients.

In 1960, Weston published an account of examples of various activities that would be appropriate to meet the needs of the aggressive child, the submissive child, the autistic and the compulsive child. Again activities were chosen which were believed to address the needs of these patients. However, there is no evidence of an empirical, as opposed to an intuitive, approach in the selection of activity.

The first instance of an empirical attempt to understand activity is found in work by Niswander and Hyde (1954). They look at reasons for choice of activity in an effort to uncover what patients derived from their participation. They found that patients chose activities that were familiar, easy, or that allowed socialization.

The most sophisticated early effort to develop an empirical basis for activity analysis is a study by Smith, Barrows and Whitney (1959). They used a technique modelled on the Osgood Semantic Differential (Osgood, 1957) to discover affective meaning of nine craft activities with three patient populations. Following factor analysis, four factors were identified for each activity, i.e., appeal, potency, difficulty and cleanliness. This new knowledge was then used to suggest applications for the various crafts within a psychodynamic model. Differences were noted in the meaning attributed to the activities between the different diagnostic groups, and between patients and therapists. This latter finding confirmed the doubt expressed earlier about whether therapists could accurately analyze activities by projecting their own impressions onto them.

Allard (1964) looked at the ability of therapists to reliably rate 17 activities on seven factors related to physical and psychological demands of the activity. She hypothesized that acceptable levels of inter-rater reliability would confirm that occupational therapists employ sound judgement when analyzing activities. She found an average coefficient of reliability of .67 on the seventeen activities, with coefficients as high as .96 on the more specifically defined activities.

In 1967, Fox and Jirgal also looked at therapist reliability in activity analysis in a survey of twenty occupational therapists. Therapists were asked to rank ten activities on each of a series of 28 physical and psychological therapeutic properties. The study resulted in a listing of fifteen properties for which therapists produced a ranking of activities with Kendall coefficients of concordance of greater than .80.

In the period between 1967 and 1982, little attention was devoted in the occupational therapy literature to advancing the understanding of activity and activity analysis. Renewed interest, however, was expressed recently in a series of studies emerging out of the Boston area, examining the meaning of activity by again using the Osgood Semantic Differential technique (Osgood, 1957). The first looked at the meaning of 4 activities among normal college students, on the three dimensions of evaluation, potency and activity (Nelson, Thompson and Moore, 1982). A second study looked at the effect of personality type on response to activity, and found no significant difference between two distinct personality types on two activities (Carter, Nelson and Duncombe, 1983). Henry, Nelson and Duncombe (1984) looked at the importance of choice-making on the perception of activity. They found that the sense of power was enhanced by allowing patients free choice in activity when conducted in a group situation. Finally, Kremer, Nelson and Duncombe (1984) conducted a study to examine the meaning of three activities to a group of chronic psychiatric patients with mixed diagnoses. They showed that different activities elicited different affective responses from this client population, thus "add(ing) to our understanding of the use of activity analysis with a mental health population" (p. 527).

These more recent studies represent a shift away from the traditional intuitive approach to activity analysis, towards a more empirical conceptualization of activity. They further demonstrate the re-commitment to first principles that Shannon (1977) and Gillette and Kielhofner (1979) recommend as the best remedy to the current process of derailment. What is required now is a more detailed understanding of both the meaning of activity with specific patient groups, and the link between activity and various psychological constructs, such as effectiveness. Work with anorexics increases awareness of the inadequacy of current methods in occupational therapy for choosing activities which can remediate the sense of effectiveness.

IMPLICATIONS FOR TREATMENT AND RESEARCH WITH ANOREXICS

It is proposed that principles of treatment to remediate a sense of ineffectiveness in anorexia should follow a developmental paradigm; just as the sense of effectiveness is developed initially in the healthy child, so should it be remediated. A growth facilitating environment should be provided in occupational therapy which simulates the conditions under which the normal developmental stage occurs (Mosey, 1970). There should be opportunity for exploratory behaviour and interaction with the environment. The environment should be pliable and responsive to such interaction. Interaction should, in and of itself, be valued and respected by the therapist and positively reinforced. The environment should encourage a degree of risk-taking behaviour without fear of censure or serious consequences. Activities which are pursued should be determined by conscious choice and decision-making. The anorexic is to be aware that she is exercising her own free will and that this—and not the end result of the activity—is what matters. For the anorexic, it is not competence but the sense of personal effectiveness that needs to be remediated. It is important then, not to prescribe activity. Breines (1984) stresses the importance of choice in activity, noting that the goals must be those of the patient. She goes so far as to state that purposeful activity cannot be defined by one person for another. This statement echoes earlier views put forth by Meyer (1921) regarding the philosophy of occupational therapy, when he stated that activity was ''not a question of specific prescriptions but of opportunities'' (p. 641). The importance of choice is also noted by Burke (1977) who sees this element as important in remediating the sense of control in the physically disabled population; the principle seems equally applicable to remediation of the sense of ineffectiveness in anorexics.

Although the principle of choice can readily be adhered to in the treatment setting, it must be acknowledged that in reality, only a finite number of activities will be available from which to choose. What will these activities be? Are there qualities inherent in certain activities that can, in a real or symbolic way, provide an opportunity to develope the sense of effectiveness? Would these qualities be perceived in the same way by all people? Would there be a difference for example, in the way anorexics perceive such an activity compared to other patients, or compared to people who are well? Empirical information on the meaning of activity to anorexics is needed before further advancement can be made in this important area. It is sobering to consider Fidler's statement that although activity has been the fundamental concept in occupational therapy since its inception, we still do not know "the why, the what, the when and the how of activities" (Fidler, 1981, p. 570).

REFERENCES

Allard I (1964) Our professional judgement: Sound or haphazard. *American Journal of Occupational Therapy, 18,* 104-7.

American Psychiatric Association (1980) *Diagnostic and Statistical Manual of Mental Disorders,* Third Edition, Washington, D.C., APA.

Bandura A (1977) Self-efficacy: Toward a theory of behaviour change. *Psychological Review, 84,* 191-215.

Bemis KM (1978) Current approachs to the etiology and treatment of anorexia nervosa. *Psychological Bulletin, 85,* 593-617.

Bissell JC, Mailloux Z (1981) The use of crafts in occupational therapy for the physically disabled. *American Journal of Occupational Therapy, 35,* 369-74.

Breines E (1980) An attempt to define purposeful activity. *American Journal of Occupational Therapy, 38,* 543-544.

Bruch H (1973) *Eating Disorders.* New York: Basic Books.

Bruch H (1979) *The golden cage. The enigma of anorexia nervosa.* New York: Vintage Books.

Bruch H (1985) Four decades of eating disorders. In D.M. Garner and P.E. Garfinkel (Eds.), *Handbook of Psychotherapy for Anorexia Nervosa and Bulimia.* New York: Guilford Press.

Burke JP (1977) A clinical perspective on motivation: Pawn vs. origin. *American Journal of Occupational Therapy, 31,* 254-8.

Carter BA, Nelson DL, Duncombe LW (1983) The effect of psychological type on the mood and meaning of two collage activities. *American Journal of Occupational Therapy, 37,* 688-93.

Crisp AH, Palmer RL, Kalucy RS (1976) How common is anorexia nervosa? A prevalence study. *British Journal of Psychiatry, 218,* 549-554.

De Charms R (1968) *Personal causation.* New York: Academic Press.

Engelhardt HT (1977) Defining occupational therapy. *American Journal of Occupational Therapy, 31,* 666-72.

Fidler GS (1981) From crafts to competence. *American Journal of Occupational Therapy, 35,* 567-73.

Fidler GS (1948) Psychological evaluation of occupational therapy activities. *American Journal of Occupational Therapy, 2,* 284-87.

Fidler GS and Fidler JW (1978) Doing and becoming: Purposeful action and self actualization. *American Journal of Occupational Therapy, 32,* 8-13.

Fox and Jirgal (1967) Therapeutic properties of activities as examined by the clinical council of the Wisconsin school of Occupational Therapy. *American Journal of Occupational Therapy, 21,* 29-33.

Garfinkel PE and Garner DM (1982) *Anorexia Nervosa. A multidimensional perspective.* New York: Bruner/Mazel.

Gillette N and Kielhofner G (1979) The impact of specialization on professionalization and survival of occupational therapy. *American Journal of Occupational Therapy, 33,* 20-39.

Henry AD, Nelson DL and Duncombe L (1984) Choice-making in group and individual activities. *American Journal of Occupational Therapy, 38,* 245-51.

Hinojosa J, Sabari J and Rosenfeld MS (1983) Position paper: Purposeful activity. *American Journal of Occupational Therapy, 37,* 805-6.

Jones DL, Fox MM, Babigan HM and Hutton HE (1980) Epidemiology of anorexia nervosa in Monroe County, New York: 1960-1976. *Psychosomatic Medicine, 42,* 551-558.

Kielhofner G (1978) General systems theory. Implications for theory and action in occupational therapy. *American Journal of Occupational Therapy, 32,* 637-645.

Kielhofner G and Burke JP (1977) Occupational therapy after sixty years. *American Journal of Occupational Therapy, 31,* 675-89.

Kremer ERH, Nelson DL and Duncombe LW (1984) Effects of selected activities on affective meaning in psychiatric patients. *American Journal of Occupational Therapy, 38,* 522-8.

Meyer A (1921)

Meyer A (1977) The philosophy of occupational therapy. *American Journal of Occupational Therapy, 31,* 641.

Mosey AC (1970) *Three frames of reference for mental health.* Thorofare, New Jersey: Charles B. Slack.

Nelson DL, Thompson G and Moore JA (1982) Identification of factors of affective meaning in four selected activities. *American Journal of Occupational Therapy, 36,* 381-7.

Niswander PD and Hyde RW (1954) The value of crafts in psychiatry occupational therapy. *American Journal of Occupational Therapy, 8,* 104-6.

Osgood CE, Suci GJ and Tannenbaum PH (1957) *The measurement of meaning.* Urbana: University of Illinois Publ.

Piaget J (1952) *The origins of intelligence in children.* New York: W.W. Norton.

Reilly M (1962) Occupational therapy can be one of the great ideas of 20th century medicine. *American Journal of Occupational Therapy, 16,* 1-9.

Shannon PD (1977) The derailment of occupational therapy. *American Journal of Occupational Therapy, 31,* 229-34.

Smith PA, Barrows HS and Whitney JN (1959) Psychological attributes of occupational therapy crafts. *American Journal of Occupational Therapy, 8,* 16-26.

Taber, F, Baron S and Blackwell A (1953) A study of task directed and free choice groups. *American Journal of Occupational Therapy, 7,* 118-23.

Weston DL (1960) Therapeutic crafts. *American Journal of Occupational Therapy, 14,* 121, 2, 33.

White RW (1959) Motivation reconsidered. The concepts of competence. *Psychological Review, 66,* 297-333.

White RW (1971) The urge towards competence. *American Journal of Occupational Therapy, XXV,* 2782-274.

T - #0249 - 101024 - C0 - 212/152/9 [11] - CB - 9780866565417 - Gloss Lamination